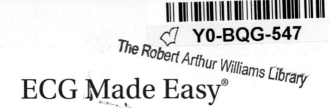

ECG Made Easy®

System requirement:

- Operating System – Windows Vista or above
- Recommended Web Browser – Google Chrome and Mozilla Firefox
- Essential plugins – Java and Flash player
    - Facing problems in viewing content – it may be your system does not have java enabled.
    - If Videos don't show up – it may be the system requires Flash player or need to manage flash setting. To learn more about flash setting click on the link in the help section.
    - You can test java and flash by using the links from the help section of the CD/DVD.

Accompanying CD/DVD-ROM is playable only in Computer and not in DVD player.

CD/DVD has Autorun function – it may take few seconds to load on your computer. If it does not works for you then follow the steps below to access the contents manually:

- Click on my computer
- Select the CD/DVD drive and click open/explore – this will show list of files in the CD/DVD
- Find and double click file – "launch.html"

CD Contents

- **The Technique of Recording an ECG.**

ECG Made Easy®

Fifth Edition

Atul Luthra
MBBS MD DNB
Diplomate National Board of Medicine
Physician, Cardiologist and Diabetologist
New Delhi, India
www.atulluthra.in
dratulluthra@gmail.com

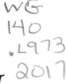
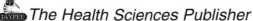*The Health Sciences Publisher*
New Delhi | London | Philadelphia | Panama

Jaypee Brothers Medical Publishers (P) Ltd

Headquarters

Jaypee Brothers Medical Publishers (P) Ltd
4838/24, Ansari Road, Daryaganj
New Delhi 110 002, India
Phone: +91-11-43574357
Fax: +91-11-43574314
Email: jaypee@jaypeebrothers.com

Overseas Offices

J.P. Medical Ltd
83 Victoria Street, London
SW1H 0HW (UK)
Phone: +44 20 3170 8910
Fax: +44 (0)20 3008 6180
Email: info@jpmedpub.com

Jaypee Medical Inc
325 Chestnut Street
Suite 412, Philadelphia, PA 19106, USA
Phone: +1 267-519-9789
Email: support@jpmedus.com

Jaypee Brothers Medical Publishers (P) Ltd
Bhotahity, Kathmandu
Nepal
Phone: +977-9741283608
Email: kathmandu@jaypeebrothers.com

Jaypee-Highlights Medical Publishers Inc
City of Knowledge, Bld. 235, 2nd Floor, Clayton
Panama City, Panama
Phone: +1 507-301-0496
Fax: +1 507-301-0499
Email: cservice@jphmedical.com

Jaypee Brothers Medical Publishers (P) Ltd
17/1-B Babar Road, Block-B, Shaymali
Mohammadpur, Dhaka-1207
Bangladesh
Mobile: +08801912003485
Email: jaypeedhaka@gmail.com

Website: www.jaypeebrothers.com

Website: www.jaypeedigital.com

© 2017, Jaypee Brothers Medical Publishers

Inquiries for bulk sales may be solicited at: jaypee@jaypeebrothers.com

ECG Made Easy®

First Edition : 1998
Second Edition : 2004
Third Edition : 2007
Fourth Edition : 2012
Fifth Edition : **2017**

ISBN: 978-93-86150-21-9

Printed at Sanat Printers

Dedicated to

My Parents
Ms Prem Luthra
and
Mr Prem Luthra
who guide and bless me
from heaven

PREFACE

The imaging techniques of contemporary 'high-tech' cardiology have failed to eclipse the primacy of the 12-lead ECG in the initial evaluation of heart disease. This simple, cost-effective and readily available diagnostic modality continues to intrigue and baffle the clinician as much as it confuses the student. A colossal volume of literature on understanding ECG bears testimony to this fact.

This book is yet another humble attempt to bring the subject of ECG closer to the hearts of students and clinicians in a simple and concise form. As the chapters unfold, the subject gradually evolves from basics to therapeutics. Although emphasis is on ECG diagnosis, causation of abnormalities and their clinical relevance are briefly mentioned too. This should help students preparing for their examinations without having to search through voluminous textbooks.

While some arrhythmias are harmless, others are ominous and life-threatening. The clinical challenge lies in knowing the cause of an arrhythmia, its significance, differential diagnosis and practical aspects of management. Therefore, seemingly similar cardiac rhythms are discussed together under individual chapter headings. Medical students, resident doctors, nurses and technicians will find this format particularly useful.

I have thoroughly enjoyed the experience of writing this book and found teaching as pleasurable as learning. Since the scope for further refinement always remains, it is a privilege to bring out the vastly improved 5th edition of *ECG Made Easy*. Your appreciation, comments and criticisms are bound to spur me on even further.

Atul Luthra

ACKNOWLEDGMENTS

I am extremely grateful to:

- My school teachers who helped me to acquire good command over the English language.
- My professors at medical college who taught me the science and art of electrocardiography.
- My heart patients whose cardiograms stimulated my brain cells to make me a wiser clinician.
- Authors of textbooks on clinical cardiology to which I referred liberally, while preparing the manuscript.
- My esteemed readers of earlier editions, whose generous appreciation and valuable criticism keep me going.
- My soulmate Reena who is a source of constant inspiration to me and appreciates all my academic pursuits.
- Shri Jitendar P Vij (Group Chairman), Mr Ankit Vij (Group President) and Mr Tarun Duneja (Director–Publishing) of M/s Jaypee Brothers Medical Publishers (P) Ltd, New Delhi, India, who repose their unflinching faith in me and my writing ability.

CONTENTS

Nomenclature of ECG Deflections

ELECTROCARDIOGRAM

The electrocardiogram (ECG) provides a graphic depiction of the electrical forces generated by the heart. The ECG graph appears as a series of deflections and waves produced by each cardiac cycle.

Before going on to the genesis of individual deflections and their terminology, it would be worthwhile mentioning certain important facts about the direction and magnitude of ECG waves and the activation pattern of myocardium.

Direction

- By convention, a deflection above the baseline or isoelectric (neutral) line is a positive deflection while one below the isoelectric line is a negative deflection **(Fig. 1.1A)**
- The direction of a deflection depends upon two factors namely, the direction of spread of the electrical force and the location of the recording electrode
- In other words, an electrical impulse moving towards an electrode creates a positive deflection while an impulse moving away from an electrode creates a negative deflection **(Fig. 1.1B)**. Let us see this example.

We know that the sequence of electrical activation is such that the interventricular septum is first activated from left to

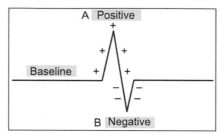

Fig. 1.1A: Direction of the deflection on ECG. (A) Above the baseline—positive deflection; (B) Below the baseline—negative deflection

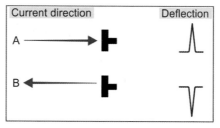

Fig. 1.1B: Effect of current direction on polarity of deflection. (A) Towards the electrode—upright deflection; (B) Away from electrode—inverted deflection

right followed by activation of the left ventricular free wall from the endocardial to epicardial surface.

If an electrode is placed over the right ventricle, it records an initial positive deflection representing septal activation towards it, followed by a major negative deflection that denotes free wall activation away from it **(Fig. 1.2)**.

If, however, the electrode is placed over the left ventricle, it records an initial negative deflection representing septal activation away from it, followed by a major positive deflection that denotes free wall activation towards it **(Fig. 1.2)**.

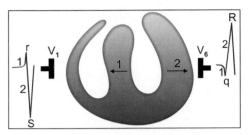

Fig. 1.2: Septal (1) and left ventricular (2) activation. As seen from lead V_1 (rS pattern); As seen from lead V_6 (qR pattern)

Magnitude

- The height of a positive deflection and the depth of a negative deflection are measured vertically from the baseline. This vertical amplitude of the deflection is a measure of its voltage in millimeters **(Fig. 1.3A)**
- The magnitude of a deflection depends upon the quantum of the electrical forces generated by the heart and the extent to which they are transmitted to the recording electrode on the body surface. Let us see these examples:
  - ⟶ Since the ventricle has a far greater muscle mass than the atrium, ventricular complexes are larger than atrial complexes
  - ⟶ When the ventricular wall undergoes thickening (hypertrophy), the ventricular complexes are larger than normal
  - ⟶ If the chest wall is thick, the ventricular complexes are smaller than normal since the fat or muscle intervenes between the myocardium and the recording electrode **(Fig. 1.3B)**.

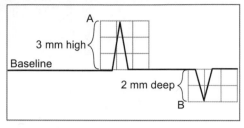

Fig. 1.3A: Magnitude of the ECG deflection. (A) Positive deflection—height; (B) Negative deflection—depth

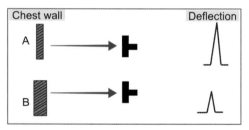

Fig. 1.3B: Effect of chest wall on magnitude of deflection. (A) Thin chest—tall deflection; (B) Thick chest—small deflection

Activation

- Activation of the atria occurs longitudinally by contiguous spread of electrical forces from one myocyte to the other. On the other hand, activation of the ventricles occurs transversely by spread of electrical forces from the endocardial surface (surface facing ventricular cavity) to the epicardial surface (outer surface) **(Fig. 1.4).**

  Therefore, atrial activation can reflect atrial enlargement (and not atrial hypertrophy) while ventricular activation can reflect ventricular hypertrophy (and not ventricular enlargement).

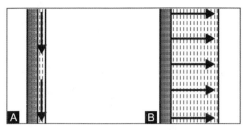

Fig. 1.4: Direction of myocardial activation in atrium and ventricle. (A) Atrial muscle—longitudinal, from one myocyte to other; (B) Ventricular—transverse, endocardium to epicardium

ELECTROPHYSIOLOGY

The ECG graph consists of a series of deflections or waves. The distances between sequential waves on the time axis are termed as intervals. Portions of the isoelectric line (baseline) between successive waves are termed as segments.

In order to understand the genesis of deflections and the significance of intervals and segments, it would be worthwhile understanding certain basic electrophysiological principles.

- Anatomically speaking, the heart is a four-chambered organ. But in the electrophysiological sense, it is actually two-chambered. As per the "dual-chamber" concept, the chambers of the heart are the biatrial chamber and the biventricular chamber **(Fig. 1.5).** This is because the atria are activated together and the ventricles too contact synchronously. Therefore, on the ECG, atrial activation is represented by a single wave and ventricular activation by a single wave-complex
- In the resting state, the myocyte membrane bears a negative charge on the inner side. When stimulated by an electrical impulse, the charge is altered by an influx of calcium ions across the cell membrane.

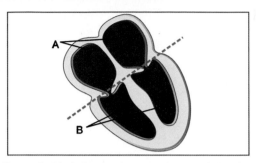

Fig. 1.5: The "dual-chamber" concept. (A) Biatrial chamber;
(B) Biventricular chamber

This results in coupling of actin and myosin filaments and muscle contraction. The spread of electrical impulse through the myocardium is known as depolarization **(Fig. 1.6)**

- Once the muscle contraction is completed, there is efflux of potassium ions, in order to restore the resting state of the cell membrane. This results in uncoupling of actin and myosin filaments and muscle relaxation. The return of the myocardium to its resting electrical state is known as repolarization **(Fig. 1.6)**
- Depolarization and repolarization occur in the atrial muscle as well as in the ventricular myocardium. The wave of excitation is synchronized so that the atria and the ventricles contract and relax in a rhythmic sequence
- Atrial depolarization is followed by atrial repolarization which is nearly synchronous with ventricular depolarization and finally ventricular repolarization occurs
- We must appreciate that depolarization and repolarization of the heart muscle are electrical events, while cardiac contraction (systole) and relaxation (diastole) constitute mechanical events

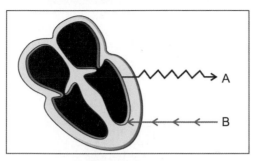

Fig. 1.6: The spread of impulse. (A) Depolarization; (B) Repolarization

- However, it is true that depolarization just precedes systole and repolarization is immediately followed by diastole.
- The electrical impulse that initiates myocardial depolarization and contraction originates from a group of cells that comprise the pacemaker of the heart
- The normal pacemaker is the sinoatrial (SA) node, situated in the upper portion of the right atrium **(Fig. 1.7)**
- From the SA node, the electrical impulse spreads to the right atrium through three intra-atrial pathways while the Bachmann's bundle carries the impulse to the left atrium
- Having activated the atria, the impulse enters the atrioventricular (AV) node situated at the AV junction on the lower part of the interatrial septum. The brief delay of the impulse at the AV node allows time for the atria to empty the blood they contain into their respective ventricles.

After the AV nodal delay, the impulse travels to the ventricles through a specialized conduction system called the bundle of His. The His bundle primarily divides into two bundle branches, a right bundle branch (RBB) which traverses the right ventricle and a left bundle branch (LBB) that traverses the left ventricle **(Fig. 1.7)**.

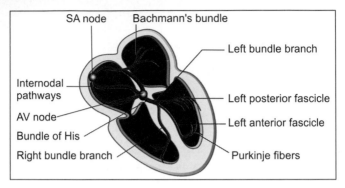

Fig. 1.7: The electrical 'wiring' network of the heart

A small septal branch originates from the left bundle branch to activate the interventricular septum from left to right. The left bundle branch further divides into a left posterior fascicle and a left anterior fascicle.

The posterior fascicle is a broad band of fibers which spreads over the posterior and inferior surfaces of the left ventricle. The anterior fascicle is a narrow band of fibers, which spreads over the anterior and superior surfaces of the left ventricle **(Fig. 1.7).**

Having traversed the bundle branches, the impulse finally passes into their terminal ramifications called Purkinje fibers. These Purkinje fibers traverse the thickness of the myocardium to activate the entire myocardial mass from the endocardial surface to the epicardial surface.

DEFLECTIONS

The ECG graph consists of a series of deflections or waves. Each electrocardiographic deflection has been arbitrarily assigned a letter of the alphabet. Accordingly, a sequence of wave that represents a single cardiac cycle is sequentially termed as P Q R S T and U **(Fig. 1.8A).**

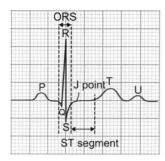

Fig. 1.8A: The normal ECG deflections

By convention, P, T and U waves are always denoted by capital letters while the Q, R and S waves can be represented by either a capital letter or a small letter depending upon their relative or absolute magnitude. Large waves (over 5 mm) are assigned capital letters Q, R and S while small waves (under 5 mm) are assigned small letters q, r and s.

The entire QRS complex is viewed as one unit, since it represents ventricular depolarization. The positive deflection is always called the R wave. The negative deflection before the R wave is the Q wave while the negative deflection after the R wave is the S wave **(Fig. 1.8B)**.

Relatively speaking, a small q followed by a tall R is labeled as qR complex while a large Q followed by a small r is labeled as Qr complex. Similarly, a small r followed by a deep S is termed as rS complex, while a tall R followed by a small s is termed as Rs complex **(Fig. 1.9)**.

Two other situations are worth mentioning. If a QRS deflection is totally negative without an ensuing positivity, it is termed as a QS complex.

Secondly, if the QRS complex reflects two positive waves, the second positive wave is termed as R' and accordingly, the complex is termed as rSR' or RsR' depending upon magnitude

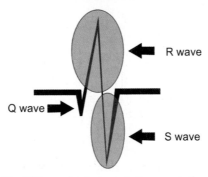

Fig. 1.8B: The QRS complex is one unit. Q wave—before R wave;
S wave—after R wave

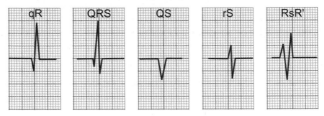

Fig. 1.9: Various configurations of the QRS complex

of the positive (r or R) wave and the negative (s or S) wave
(Fig. 1.9).

Significance of ECG Deflections

- P wave :   Produced by atrial depolarization.
- QRS complex :   Produced by ventricular depolarization.
                    It consists of:
    - Q wave :   First negative deflection before R wave.
    - R wave :   First positive deflection after Q wave.
    - S wave :   First negative deflection after R wave.
- T wave :   Produced by ventricular repolarization.
- U wave :   Produced by Purkinje repolarization
                    (Fig. 1.10).

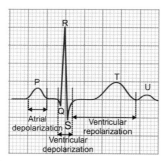

Fig. 1.10: Depolarization and repolarization depicted as deflections
(Note: Atrial repolarization is buried in the QRS complex)

Within ventricular repolarization, the ST segment is the plateau phase and the T wave is the rapid phase.

You would be wondering where is atrial repolarization. Well, it is represented by the Ta wave which occurs just after the P wave. The Ta wave is generally not seen on the ECG as it coincides with (lies buried in) the larger QRS complex.

INTERVALS

During analysis of an ECG graph, the distances between certain waves are relevant in order to establish a temporal relationship between sequential events during a cardiac cycle. Since the distance between waves is expressed on a time axis, these distances are termed as ECG intervals. The following ECG intervals are clinically important.

PR Interval

The PR interval is measured from the onset of the P wave to the beginning of the QRS complex **(Fig. 1.11)**. Although the term PR interval is in vogue, actually, PQ interval would be more appropriate. Note that the duration of the P wave is included in the measurement.

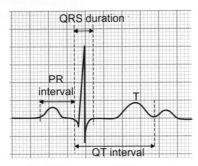

Fig. 1.11: The normal ECG intervals

We know that the P wave represents atrial depolarization while the QRS complex represents ventricular depolarization. Therefore, it is easy to comprehend that the PR interval is an expression of atrioventricular conduction time.

This includes the time for atrial depolarization, conduction delay in the AV node and the time required for the impulse to traverse the ventricular conduction system before ventricular depolarization ensues.

QT Interval

The QT interval is measured from the onset of the Q wave to the end of the T wave **(Fig. 1.11)**. If it is measured to the end of the U wave, it is termed QU interval. Note that the duration of the QRS complex, the length of the ST segment and the duration of the T wave are included in the measurement.

We know that the QRS complex represents ventricular depolarization while the T wave represents ventricular repolarization. Therefore, it is easy to comprehend that the QT interval is an expression of total duration of ventricular systole.

Since the U wave represents Purkinje system repolarization, the QU interval in addition takes into account the time taken for the ventricular Purkinje system to repolarize.

SEGMENTS

The magnitude and direction of an ECG deflection is expressed in relation to a baseline, which is referred to as the isoelectric line. The main isoelectric line is the period of electrical inactivity that intervenes between successive cardiac cycles during which no deflections are observed.

It lies between the termination of the T wave (or U wave, if seen) of one cardiac cycle and onset of the P wave of the next cardiac cycle. However, two other segments of the isoelectric line that occur between the waves of a single cardiac cycle, are clinically important.

PR Segment

The PR segment is that portion of the isoelectric line which intervenes between the termination of the P wave and the onset of the QRS complex **(Fig. 1.12).** It represents conduction delay in the atrioventricular node. Note carefully that the

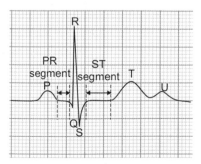

Fig. 1.12: The normal ECG segments

length of the PR segment does not include the width of the P wave, while the duration of the PR interval does include the P wave width.

ST Segment

The ST segment is that portion of the isoelectric line which intervenes between the termination of the S wave and the onset of the T wave **(Fig. 1.12).** It represents the plateau phase of ventricular repolarization. The point at which the QRS complex ends and the ST segment begins is termed the junction point or J point.

CHAPTER

2

Electrocardiographic Leads

ELECTROCARDIOGRAPHIC LEADS

During activation of the myocardium, electrical forces or action potentials are propagated in various directions. These electrical forces can be picked up from the surface of the body by means of electrodes and recorded in the form of an electrocardiogram.

A pair of electrodes, that consists of a positive and a negative electrode constitutes an electrocardiographic lead. Each lead is oriented to record electrical forces as viewed from one aspect of the heart.

The position of these electrodes can be changed so that different leads are obtained. The angle of electrical activity recorded changes with each lead. Several angles of recording provide a detailed perspective the heart.

There are twelve conventional ECG lead placements that constitute the routine 12-lead ECG **(Fig. 2.1)**.

The 12 ECG leads are:
- Limb leads or extremity leads—six in number
- Chest leads or precordial leads—six in number.

LIMB LEADS

The limb leads are derived from electrodes placed on the limbs. An electrode is placed on each of the three limbs,

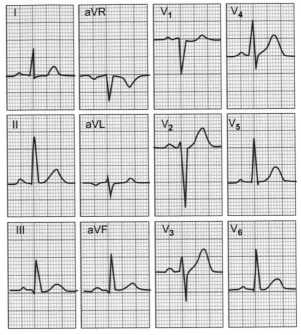

Fig. 2.1: Conventional 12-lead electrocardiogram

namely right arm, left arm and left leg. The right leg electrode acts as the grounding electrode **(Fig. 2.2A).**

- Standard limb leads—three in number
- Augmented limb leads—three in number.

Standard Limb Leads

The standard limb leads obtain a graph of the electrical forces as recorded between two limbs at a time. Therefore, the standard limb leads are also called bipolar leads. In these leads, one limb carries a positive electrode and the other limb carries a negative electrode. There are three standard limb leads **(Fig. 2.3):**

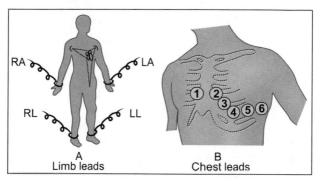

Fig. 2.2: Electrode placement for ECG recording

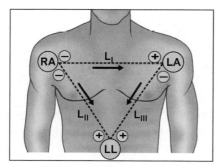

Fig. 2.3: Three standard limb leads—L_I, L_{II} and L_{III}

- Lead L_I
- Lead L_{II}
- Lead L_{III}

Lead	Positive electrode	Negative electrode
I	LA	RA
II	LL	RA
III	LL	LA

Augmented Limb Leads

The augmented limb leads obtain a graph of the electrical forces as recorded from one limb at a time. Therefore, the augmented limb leads are also called unipolar leads. In these leads, one limb carries a positive electrode, while a central terminal represents the negative pole which is actually at zero potential. There are three augmented limb leads **(Fig. 2.4):**

- Lead aVR (Right arm)
- Lead aVL (Left arm)
- Lead aVF (Foot left).

Lead	Positive electrode
aVR	RA
aVL	LA
aVF	LL

Note:

Inadvertent swapping of the leads for left and right arms (reversed arm electrodes) produces what is known as "technical" dextrocardia. The effects of arm electrode reversal on the limb leads are:

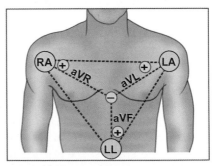

Fig. 2.4: Three unipolar limb leads—aVR, aVL and aVF

- Mirror image inversion of L_I
- aVR exchanged with aVL
- L_{II} exchanged with L_{III}
- No change in lead aVF.

This is distinguished from true mirror-image dextrocardia by the fact that chest leads are normal.

CHEST LEADS

The chest leads are obtained from electrodes placed on the precordium in designated areas. An electrode can be placed on six different positions on the left side of the chest, each position representing one lead **(Fig. 2.2B)**. Accordingly, there are six chest leads namely:

- Lead V_1 :   Over the fourth intercostal space, just to the right of sternal border
- Lead V_2 :   Over the fourth intercostal space, just to the left of sternal border
- Lead V_3 :   Over a point midway between V_2 and V_4 (see V_4 below)
- Lead V_4 :   Over the fifth intercostal space in the mid-clavicular line
- Lead V_5 :   Over the anterior axillary line, at the same level as lead V_4
- Lead V_6 :   Over the midaxillary line, at the same level as leads V_4 and V_5.

Note:

Sometimes, the chest leads are obtained from electrodes placed on the right side of the chest. The right-sided chest leads are V_{1R}, V_{2R}, V_{3R}, V_{4R}, V_{5R} and V_{6R}. These leads are mirror images of the standard left-sided chest leads.

- V_{1R} :   4th intercostal space to left of sternum
- V_{2R} :   4th intercostal space to right of sternum
- V_{3R} :   Point midway between V_{2R} and V_{4R}

- V_{4R} : 5th intercostal space in midclavicular line, and so on.

The right-sided chest leads are useful in cases of:
- True mirror-image dextrocardia
- Acute inferior wall myocardial infarction (to diagnose right ventricular infarction).

LEAD ORIENTATION

We have thus seen that the 12-lead ECG consists of the following 12 leads recorded in succession:

L_I, L_{II}, L_{III}, aVR, aVL, aVF, V_1, V_2, V_3, V_4, V_5, V_6

Since the left ventricle is the dominant and clinically the most important chamber of the heart, it needs to be assessed in detail. The left ventricle can be viewed from different angles, each with a specific set of leads. The leads with respect to different regions of the left ventricle, are shown in **Table 2.1**.

EINTHOVEN TRIANGLE

We have seen that the standard limb leads are recorded from two limbs at a time, one carrying the positive electrode and the

TABLE 2.1: Region of left ventricle represented on ECG

ECG leads	Region of left ventricle
V_1, V_2	Septal
V_3, V_4	Anterior
V_5, V_6	Lateral
V_1 to V_4	Anteroseptal
V_3 to V_6	Anterolateral
L_I, aVL	High lateral
L_{II}, L_{III}, aVF	Inferior

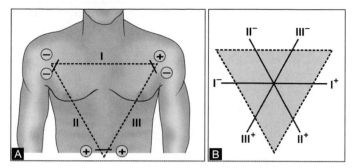

Fig. 2.5: (A) The Einthoven triangle of limb leads; (B) The triaxial reference system

other, the negative electrode. The three standard limb leads (L_I, L_{II}, L_{III}) can be seen to form an equilateral triangle with the heart at the center. This triangle is called the *Einthoven triangle* **(Fig. 2.5A)**.

To facilitate the graphic representation of electrical forces, the three limbs of the Einthoven triangle can be redrawn in such a way that the three leads they represent bisect each other and pass through a common central point. This produces a triaxial reference system with each axis separated by 60° from the other, the lead polarity (+ or –) and direction remaining the same **(Fig. 2.5B)**.

We have also seen that the augmented limb leads are recorded from one limb at a time, the limb carrying the positive electrode and the negative pole being represented by the central point. The three augmented limb leads (aVR, aVL, aVF) can be seen to form another triaxial reference system with each axis being separated by 60° from one other **(Fig. 2.6A)**.

When this triaxial system of unipolar leads is superimposed on the triaxial system of limb leads, we can derive a hexaxial reference system with each axis being separated by 30° from the other **(Fig. 2.6B)**.

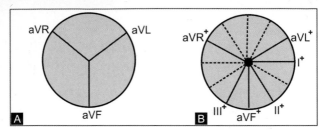

Fig. 2.6: (A) Triaxial reference system from unipolar leads; (B) Hexaxial system from unipolar and limb leads

Note carefully that each of the six leads retains its polarity (positive and negative poles) and orientation (lead direction). The hexaxial reference system concept is important in determining the major direction of the heart's electrical forces. As we shall see later, this is what we call the electrical axis of the QRS complex.

3

Electrocardiography Grid and Normal Values

ELECTROCARDIOGRAPHY GRID

The electrocardiography paper is made in such a way that it is thermosensitive. Therefore, the ECG is recorded by movement of the tip of a heated stylus over the moving paper.

The ECG paper is available as a roll of 20 or 30 meters, which when loaded into the ECG machine moves at a predetermined speed of 25 mm per second.

The ECG paper is marked like a graph, consisting of horizontal and vertical lines. There are fine lines marked 1 mm apart while every fifth line is marked boldly. Therefore, the bold lines are placed 5 mm apart **(Fig. 3.1).** Time is measured along the horizontal axis in seconds, while voltage is measured along the vertical axis in millivolts.

During ECG recording, the usual paper speed is 25 mm per second. This means that 25 small squares are covered in one second. In other words, the width of 1 small square is 1/25 or 0.04 seconds and the width of 1 large square is 0.04 × 5 or 0.2 seconds. Therefore, the width of an ECG deflection or the duration of an ECG interval is the number of small squares it occupies on the horizontal axis multiplied by 0.04 **(Fig. 3.1).** Accordingly, 2 small squares represent 0.08 seconds, 3 small squares represent 0.12 seconds and 6 small squares represent 0.24 seconds.

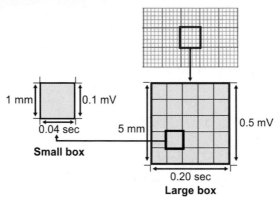

Fig. 3.1: The enlarged illustration of the electrocardiography paper. 1 small square = 1 mm; 5 small squares = 1 big square; Vertically, 1 small square = 0.1 mV. 5 of them = 0.5 mV; Horizontally, 1 small square = 0.04 sec. 5 of them = 0.2 sec

Normally, the ECG machine is standardized in such a way that a 1 millivolt signal from the machine produces a 10 millimeter vertical deflection. In other words, each small square on the vertical axis represents 0.1 mV and each large square represents 0.5 mV.

Therefore, the height of a positive deflection (above the baseline) or the depth of a negative deflection (below the baseline) is the number of small squares it occupies on the vertical axis multiplied by 0.1 mV **(Fig. 3.1).** Accordingly, 3 small squares represent 0.3 mV, 1 large square represents 0.5 mV and 6 small squares represent 0.6 mV.

Similarly, the degree of elevation (above the baseline) or depression (below the baseline) of segment is expressed in number of small squares (millimeters) of segment elevation or segment depression in relation to the isoelectric line.

NORMAL ECG VALUES

Normal P Wave

The P wave is a small rounded wave produced by atrial depolarization. In fact, it reflects the sum of right and left atrial activation, the right preceding the left, since the pacemaker is located in the right atrium **(Fig. 3.2A)**.

The P wave is normally upright in most of the ECG leads with two exceptions. In lead aVR, it is inverted along with inversion of the QRS complex and the T wave, since the direction of atrial activation is away from this lead.

In lead V_1, it is generally biphasic that is upright but with a small terminal negative deflection, representing left atrial activation in a reverse direction.

Normally, the P wave has a single peak without a gap or notch between the right and left atrial components. A normal P wave meets the following criteria:
- Less than 2.5 mm (0.25 mV) in height
- Less than 2.5 mm (0.10 second) in width **(Fig. 3.2B)**.

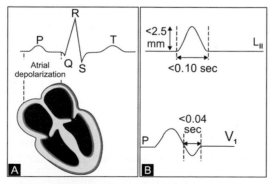

Fig. 3.2: (A) Atrial depolarization; (B) The normal P wave

Normal QRS Complex

The QRS complex is the major positive deflection on the ECG produced by ventricular depolarization. In fact, it represents the timing and sequence of synchronized depolarization of the right and left ventricles.

The Q wave is not visible in all ECG leads. Physiological Q waves may be observed in leads L_I, aVL, V_5 and V_6 where they represent initial activation of the interventricular septum in a direction opposite to the direction of activation of the main left ventricular mass.

A physiological Q wave meets the following criteria:

- Less than 0.04 second in width
- Less than 25 percent of R wave **(Fig. 3.3A).**

The leads in which physiological Q waves appear depends upon the direction towards which the main mass of the left ventricle is oriented.

If the left ventricle is directed towards the lateral leads (horizontal heart), Q waves appear in leads L_I, aVL, V_5 and V_6 **(Fig. 3.3B).** If it is directed towards the inferior leads (vertical heart), Q waves appear in leads L_{II}, L_{III} and aVF.

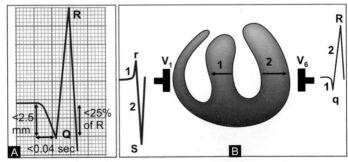

Fig. 3.3: (A) The normal Q wave; (B) Septal depolarization (1)

The R wave is the major positive deflection of the QRS complex. It is upright in most leads, except in lead aVR where the P wave and T wave are also inverted.

In the limb leads, R wave voltage is normally atleast 5 mm while in the precordial leads, R wave voltage exceeds 10 mm. Under normal circumstances, the R wave voltage gradually increases as we move from lead V_1 to lead V_6. This is known as normal R wave progression in precordial leads. Normally, the R wave amplitude does not exceed 0.4 mV (4 mm) in lead V_1 where it reflects septal activation, and does not exceed 2.5 mV (25 mm) in lead V_6 where it reflects left ventricular activation **(Fig. 3.4A)**.

The r wave is smaller than the S wave in lead V_1 and the R wave is taller than the s wave in lead V_6. The S wave is the negative deflection that follows the R wave, representing the terminal portion of ventricular depolarization.

In lead V_1, the S wave reflects left ventricular activation while in lead V_6 the s wave reflects right ventricular activation. Normally, the S wave magnitude is greater than the r wave height in lead V_1 and the s wave is smaller than the R wave in lead V_6. The normal s wave voltage in lead V_6 does not exceed 0.7 mV.

The QRS complex represents depolarization of the total ventricular muscle. The relative amplitude of the R wave and S wave in a particular lead reflects the relative contributions of the right and left ventricles.

For instance in lead V_1, the r wave is smaller than the S wave while in lead V_6 the s wave is smaller than the R wave. The duration of the QRS complex is the total time taken for both ventricles to be depolarized. Since the right and left ventricles are depolarized in a synchronous fashion, the normal QRS complex is narrow, has a sharp peak and measures less than 0.08 second (2 mm) on the horizontal axis **(Fig. 3.4B)**.

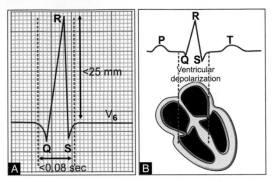

Fig. 3.4: (A) The normal QRS complex; (B) Ventricular depolarization

Normal T Wave

The T wave is a large rounded wave produced by the rapid phase of ventricular repolarization **(Fig. 3.5).** The T wave is normally upright in most leads with certain exceptions.

It is invariably inverted in lead aVR along with inversion of the P wave and QRS complex. It is often inverted in lead V_1, occasionally in lead V_2, V_3 and sometimes in lead L_{III}. The normal T wave is taller in lead V_6 than in lead V_1. The amplitude of the normal T wave does not generally exceed 5 mm in the limb leads and 10 mm in the precordial leads.

Normal U Wave

The U wave is a small rounded wave produced by slow and late repolarization of the intraventricular Purkinje system, after the main ventricular mass has been repolarized **(Fig. 3.5).**

It is often difficult to notice the U wave but when seen, it is best appreciated in the precordial leads V_2 to V_4. The U wave is more easy to recognize when the Q-T interval is short or the

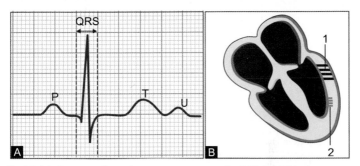

Fig. 3.5: (A) The normal T and U waves as seen on the ECG; (B) (1) T wave—ventricular mass repolarization, (2) U wave—Purkinje system repolarization

heart rate is slow, in which conditions it is clearly separated from the preceding T wave and the P wave of the following beat respectively.

The normal U wave is upright and it is normally much smaller than the T wave, which it follows.

Normal PR Interval

The PR interval is measured on the horizontal axis from the onset of the P wave to the beginning of the QRS complex, irrespective of whether it begins with a Q wave or a R wave **(Fig. 3.6).**

Since, the P wave represents atrial depolarization and the QRS complex represents ventricular depolarization, the PR interval is a measure of the atrioventricular (AV) conduction time.

The AV conduction time includes time for atrial depolarization, conduction delay in the AV node and time required for the impulse to traverse the conduction system before ventricular depolarization begins.

The normal PR interval is in the range of 0.12 to 0.20 second, depending upon the heart rate. It is prolonged at slow heart rates and shortened at fast heart rates. The PR interval tends to be slightly shorter in children (upper limit 0.18 second) and slightly longer in elderly persons (upper limit 0.22 second).

Normal QT Interval

The QT interval is measured on the horizontal axis from the onset of the Q wave to the end of the T wave **(Fig. 3.6).**

Since, the QRS complex represents ventricular depolarization and the T wave represents ventricular repolarization, QT interval denotes the total duration of ventricular systole. The QT interval includes the duration of QRS complex, the length of ST segment and the width of the T wave. The normal QT interval is in the range of 0.35 to 0.43 second or 0.39 $\pm$ 0.04 second. The QT interval depends upon three variables namely age, sex and heart rate. The QT interval tends to be shorter in young individuals and longer in the elderly. It is normally, slightly shorter in females, the upper limit being 0.42 second. The QT interval shortens at fast heart rates and lengthens at slow heart rates.

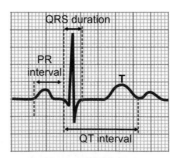

Fig. 3.6: The normal ECG intervals

Therefore, for proper interpretation, the QT interval must be corrected for the heart rate. The corrected QT interval is known as the QTc interval. The QTc interval is determined using the formula:

$$Q{-}Tc = \frac{Q-T}{\sqrt{R-R}}$$

where, QT is the measured QT interval, and $\sqrt{RR}$ is the square root of the measured RR interval.

Since, the RR interval at a heart rate of 60 is 25 mm or 1 second (25×0.04 second = 1 second), the QTc interval is equal to the QT interval at a heart rate of 60 per minute.

Normal PR Segment

The portion of the baseline (isoelectric line), which intervenes between the termination of the P wave and the onset of the QRS complex, is the PR segment **(Fig. 3.7)**.

Normally, it is at the same level as the main segment of the isoelectric line which intervenes between the T wave of one cycle and the P wave of the next cycle.

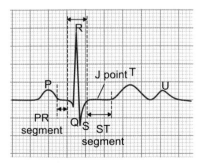

Fig. 3.7: The normal ECG segments

Normal ST Segment

The portion of the baseline (isoelectric line), which intervenes between the termination of the S wave and the onset of the T wave, is the ST segment **(Fig. 3.7).**

The beginning of the ST segment is the junction point (J point). Normally, the ST segment and the J point are in level with the main segment of the isoelectric line, which intervenes between the T wave of one cycle and the P wave of the next cycle.

4

Determination of Electrical Axis

ELECTRICAL AXIS

During activation of the heart, the electrical forces or action potentials which have been generated, are propagated in various directions. These electrical forces can be picked up from the surface of the body by means of electrodes.

Normally, over 80 percent of these forces are cancelled out by equal and opposing forces, and only the net forces remaining, are recorded. The dominant direction of these forces, which is the mean of all recorded forces constitutes the electrical axis of an electrocardiographic deflection.

Since, the QRS complex is the major deflection on the ECG, we shall confine ourselves to the QRS electrical axis.

HEXAXIAL SYSTEM

We have already seen that the three standard limb leads L_I, L_{II} and L_{III} form an equilateral triangle with the heart at its center, which is called the Einthoven triangle.

The Einthoven triangle can be redrawn in such a way that the three leads pass through a common central point. This constitutes a triaxial reference system with each axis separated from the other by 60°.

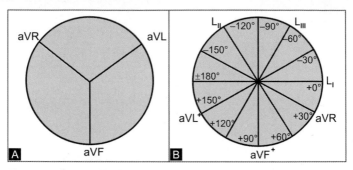

Fig. 4.1: (A) The triaxial reference system from unipolar leads; (B) The hexaxial system from unipolar and limb leads

Similarly, the three augmented limb leads can constitute another triaxial reference system **(Fig. 4.1A)**. When these two triaxial systems are superimposed on each other, we can construct a hexaxial reference system in a 360° circle, with each axis separated from the other by 30° **(Fig. 4.1B)**.

In the hexaxial system, each of the six leads maintains its own polarity and direction. The hexaxial reference system is the basis of understanding the concept of electrical axis and its determination.

QRS AXIS

Before going on to the actual determination of the QRS axis, certain basic principles have to be understood.

- The QRS axis is expressed as a degree on the hexaxial system and represents the direction of electrical forces in the frontal plane **(Fig. 4.2)**
- The net deflection in any lead is the algebraic sum of the positive and negative deflections. For instance, if in any lead, the positive deflection (R) is +6 and the negative deflection (S) is –2, the net deflection is +4

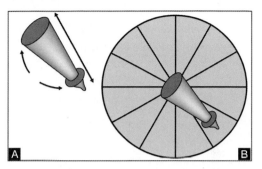

Fig. 4.2: (A) The direction and magnitude of the QRS vector;
(B) The QRS vector projected on the hexaxial system

- An electrical force that runs parallel to any lead, records the maximum deflection in that lead. An electrical force that runs obliquely to any lead, records a small deflection in that lead. An electrical force that runs perpendicular to any lead records a nil or equiphasic (positive and negative deflections equal) deflection in that lead

- As an example, if the axis is +90°, lead aVF records the maximum deflection. Lead L_I records the least deflection and the deflections in all other leads are intermediate

- If in a lead showing the maximum deflection, the major deflection is positive, the axis points towards the positive pole of that lead. Conversely, if the major deflection is negative, the axis points towards the negative pole of that particular lead

- Assume that, lead L_{II} is showing the maximum deflection say 7 mm. If it is +7, the axis is +60° while if it is –7, the axis is –120°.

DETERMINATION OF QRS AXIS

The QRS axis can be determined by several methods.

Method 1

- Find the lead with smallest or equiphasic deflection
- Determine the lead at right angles to the first lead
- See the net deflection in the second lead
- The axis is directed towards the positive or negative pole of the second lead.

Example A

- Lead with smallest deflection is aVL
- Lead at right angles to aVL is L_{II}
- Major deflection in lead L_{II} is positive axis, + 60°.

Example B

- Lead with smallest deflection is aVR
- Lead at right angles to aVR is L_{III}
- Major deflection in lead L_{III} is negative axis, –60°.

Method 2

- Find the net deflection in leads L_I and aVF, which are perpendicular to each other
- Plot the net deflection in these leads onto their respective axes, on a scale of 0 to 10
- Drop perpendicular lines from these points and plot a point where these lines intersect
- Join the center of the circle to the intersection point and extend it to the circumference
- The point on the circumference where this line intersects, is the QRS axis.

Example A

- Net deflection in L_I is +5
- Net deflection in aVF is 0 axis, 0°.

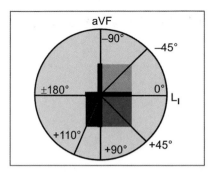

Fig. 4.3: QRS axis determined from leads LI and aVF

Example B

- Net deflection in L_I is +5
- Net deflection in aVF is –5, axis is –45° **(Fig. 4.3)**

Example C

- Net deflection in L_I is +6
- Net deflection in aVF is + 3, axis is + 30°

Method 3

For rapid and easy estimation of QRS axis, just scan the direction of the dominant deflection in leads L_I and aVF, whether positive or negative. This gives us the quadrant in which the QRS axis is located **(Table 4.1)**.

TABLE 4.1: QRS axis quadrant determined from leads L_I and aVF

Main QRS deflection		QRS axis quadrant
L_I	aVF	
+ve	+ve	0 to +90°
+ve	–ve	0 to –90°
–ve	+ve	+90 to +180°
–ve	–ve	–90 to –180°

ABNORMALITIES OF QRS AXIS

- Normal QRS axis
  –30° to + 90°
- Right axis deviation
  + 90° to + 180°
  Causes
  ⟹ Thin tall built
  ⟹ Chronic lung disease
  ⟹ Pulmonary embolism
  ⟹ Ostium secundum (ASD)
  ⟹ Right ventricular hypertrophy
  ⟹ Left posterior hemiblock
  ⟹ Lateral wall infarction
- Left axis deviation
  –30° to –90°
  Causes
  ⟹ Obese stocky built
  ⟹ Wolff-Parkinson-White (WPW) syndrome

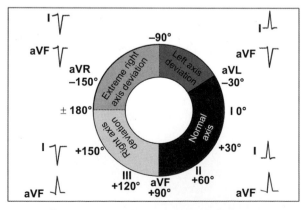

Fig. 4.4: The normal QRS axis and axis deviation

➠ Cardiac pacing
➠ Ostium primum ASD
➠ Left ventricular hypertrophy
➠ Left anterior hemiblock
➠ Inferior wall infarction

- North West QRS axis
  –90° to –180°

  Causes
  ➠ Congenital heart disease
  ➠ Left ventricular aneurysm

  Synonyms
  ➠ Indeterminate QRS axis
  ➠ Extreme right axis deviation
  ➠ No man's land **(Fig. 4.4).**

5

Determination of Heart Rate

HEART RATE

The heart rate is simply the number of heart beats per minute. In electrocardiographic terms, the heart rate is the number of cardiac cycles that occur during 60 second (1 minute) continuous recording of the ECG.

In order to calculate the heart rate from a given ECG strip, all that we have to remember is that the ECG paper moves at a speed of 25 mm per second. The rest is all deductive mathematics. Let us see how the heart rate is actually calculated.

Method 1

The ECG paper moves by 25 small squares (each small square = $1/25$ = 0.04 seconds), or by 5 large squares (each large square = 5 small squares = 0.04×5 = 0.2 seconds) in one second.

If one notes carefully, the vertical line of every fifth large square extends slightly beyond the edge of the graph paper. Therefore, the distance between two such extended lines is one second and the distance between one such line and the sixth line after it is six seconds.

We can count the number of QRS complexes in one such six second interval. Multiplying this number by ten will give us the number of QRS complexes in sixty seconds (one minute), which is the approximate heart rate.

Examples

- There are 8 QRS complexes in a 6 second interval. Heart rate is around 8 × 10 = 80 beats/minute
- There are 11 QRS complexes in a 6 second interval. Heart rate is around 11 × 10 = 110 beats/minute.

Method 2

The ECG paper moves by 25 small squares in one second. In other words, it moves by 25 × 60 = 1500 small squares in 60 seconds or one minute. If the distance between two successive ECG complexes in number of small squares is measured, the number of ECG complexes in one minute will be 1500, divided by that number. This will give us the heart rate in beats per minute **(Fig. 5.1).**

The interval between two successive P waves (PP interval) determines the atrial rate and the interval between two successive R waves (RR interval) determines the ventricular rate. During normal rhythm, the P waves and the QRS complexes track together and therefore, the heart rate

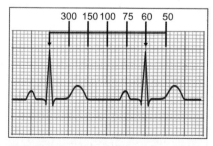

Fig. 5.1: Calculation of the heart rate from RR interval
if RR interval = 25 mm; Heart rate = 60/min

calculated by using either the PP interval or RR interval will be the same.

To measure the PP or RR interval, it is preferable to begin with a P or R wave that is superimposed on a heavy line marking of a large square. This facilitates the measurement of the interval between it and the next wave, in multiples of 5 mm (one large square = 5 small squares).

A single PP or RR interval measurement generally suffices for heart rate determination, if the heart rate is regular (equally spaced complexes). If however, the heart rate is irregular (unequally spaced complexes), a mean of 5 or 10 PP or RR intervals is taken into account.

Examples

- The RR interval is 20 mm. Therefore, the heart rate is 1500/20 = 75 beats per minute.
- The RR interval is 12 mm. Therefore, the heart rate is 1500/12 = 125 beats per minute.

For rapid heart rate determination, certain standard R-R intervals can be memorized **(Table 5.1)**.

We see that the normal RR interval ranges from 15 to 25 mm, representing a heart rate of 60–100 beats per minute. A short RR interval (less than 15 mm) denotes tachycardia

TABLE 5.1: Determining the heart rate from RR interval

RR interval	Heart rate
10 mm	1500/10 = 150
12 mm	1500/12 = 125
15 mm	1500/15 = 100
20 mm	1500/20 = 75
25 mm	1500/25 = 60
30 mm	1500/30 = 50

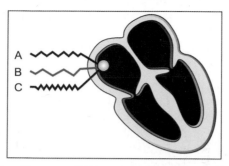

Fig. 5.2: Variation of heart rate: (A) Normal rate; (B) Bradycardia; (C) Tachycardia

(heart rate >100) and a long RR interval (more than 25 mm) denotes bradycardia (heart rate <60) **(Fig. 5.2)**.

The heart rate range can also be rapidly assessed from the range of RR interval. For instance:

• If the RR interval is 10–15 mm, the heart rate is 100–150 per minute

• If the RR interval is 15–20 mm, the heart rate is 75–100 per minute

• If the RR interval is 20–25 mm, the heart rate is 60–75 per minute.

For a more precise determination of the heart rate, we can use a reference, like the one given below **(Fig. 5.3)**.

HEART RHYTHM

The rhythm of the heart can be classified on the basis of the following criteria:

• Rate of impulse origin

• Focus of impulse origin

• Pattern of rhythm regularity

• Atrioventricular relationship.

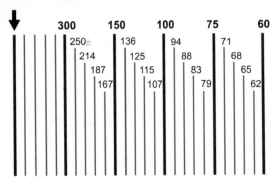

Fig. 5.3: Precise determination of the heart rate

Heart Rate

The normal heart rate varies from 60 to 100 beats per minute. A cardiac rhythm at a rate less than 60 beats per minute constitutes bradycardia. A cardiac rhythm at a rate exceeding 100 beats per minute constitutes tachycardia.

We have seen that the PP interval determines the atrial rate and the RR interval determines the ventricular rate. Normally, the PP and RR intervals are identical and the atrial rate is the same as the ventricular rate. However, under certain circumstances, the atrial and ventricular rates are different and have to be determined separately.

Under normal circumstances when the cardiac rhythm is regular, the measurement of a single RR interval suffices for heart rate determination as the QRS complexes are equally spaced. If the cardiac rhythm is irregular, that is, the QRS complexes are not equally spaced, a mean of 5 or 10 RR intervals has to be taken.

On the basis of heart rate, any cardiac rhythm can thus be classified as:

- Normal rate (HR 60–100)
- Bradycardia (HR <60)
- Tachycardia (HR >100).

Focus of Origin

The cardiac pacemaker possesses the property of automatic generation of impulses or automaticity. The normal pacemaker is the sinoatrial node (SA node) located in the right atrium.

A cardiac rhythm originating from the SA node is called sinus rhythm. The SA node normally discharges at a rate of 60–100 beats per minute. A sinus rhythm at this rate is called normal sinus rhythm.

Besides the SA node, there are other potential pacemakers in the heart such as, in the atria, atrioventricular junction and the ventricles. They are known as ectopic or subsidiary pacemakers. The subsidiary pacemakers can discharge at a slower rate than the SA node.

For instance, an atrial or junctional pacemaker can fire 40–60 impulses per minute while a ventricular pacemaker can fire 20–40 impulses per minute. It is for this reason that the SA node governs the cardiac rhythm by silencing these subsidiary pacemakers. In other words, the subsidiary pacemakers are unable to express their inherent automaticity.

However, under two situations, a subsidiary pacemaker can govern the rhythm of the heart. The first is when impulses generated from the SA node are either insufficient (sinus bradycardia) or they get blocked (SA block) and a subsidiary pacemaker is called upon to take over the cardiac rhythm. The second is when the inherent automaticity of a subsidiary pacemaker is enhanced and it over-rules the SA node to take over the cardiac rhythm.

The former situation, in which a subsidiary automaticity focus is called upon to take over the cardiac rhythm, is called an escape rhythm. The subsidiary pacemaker, so to say, escapes overdrive suppression by the SA node and expresses its inherent automaticity. The escape rhythm is triggered when intrinsic rhythm ceases or slows down and is inhibited when patient's own rhythm resumes at a reasonable rate. The subsidiary pacemaker of an escape rhythm may be junctional or ventricular. Accordingly, an escape rhythm may be classified as:

• Junctional escape rhythm or idiojunctional rhythm
• Ventricular escape rhythm or idioventricular rhythm.

The latter situation, in which a subsidiary pacemaker undergoes enhancement of its inherent automaticity so as to overrule the SA node and take overthe cardiac rhythm, is called idiofocal tachycardia. The subsidiary pacemaker of an idiofocal tachycardia may be atrial, junctional or ventricular. Accordingly, an idiofocal tachycardia may be classified as:

• Atrial tachycardia
• Junctional tachycardia
• Ventricular tachycardia.

On the basis of focus of origin, any cardiac rhythm can thus be classified as shown in **Figure 5.4:**

• Sinus rhythm
• Atrial rhythm
• Junctional rhythm
• Ventricular rhythm.

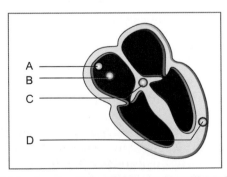

Fig. 5.4: Origin of cardiac rhythm: (A) Sinus rhythm; (B) Atrial rhythm; (C) Junctional rhythm; (D) Ventricular rhythm

Electrocardiographically, the focus of origin of a cardiac rhythm can be reasonably predicted from the morphology and relationship between P waves and QRS complexes.

In sinus rhythm, the P waves and QRS complexes are of normal morphology and normally related to each other. In other words, the P wave is upright, the PR interval is normal and the QRS complex is narrow.

In atrial rhythm, the P wave is different in morphology from the sinus wave and may be inverted due to abnormal sequence of atrial activation. The PR interval may be short, reflecting a shortened atrioventricular conduction time. However, the QRS complex retains its normal narrow configuration since intraventricular conduction of the atrial impulse proceeds as usual.

In junctional rhythm, the P wave is generally inverted and may just precede, just follow or be merged in the QRS complex. This is because the atria are activated retrogradely (from below upwards) from the junctional pacemaker and almost simultaneously with the ventricles. The QRS complexes retain their normal narrow configuration as intraventricular conduction of junctional impulses proceeds as usual.

In ventricular rhythm, either the SA node continues to activate the atria producing upright sinus P waves or the atria are activated by retrograde conduction of ventricular impulses producing inverted P waves. In both cases, the P waves are difficult to discern as the hallmark of a ventricular rhythm is wide QRS complexes in which the P waves are usually buried.

The QRS complex is wide and bizarre in a ventricular rhythm since ventricular activation occurs in a slow, random fashion through the myocardium and not in a rapid, organized fashion through the specialized conduction system (**Fig. 5.5**).

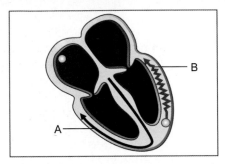

Fig. 5.5: Ventricular activation pattern: (A) Supraventricular rhythm;
(B) Ventricular rhythm

Pattern of Regularity

The normal cardiac rhythm is regular that is the interval between the different beats is the same (equally spaced QRS complexes). At times, however, the cardiac rhythm may be irregular that is the QRS complexes are not equally spaced. Irregularity of cardiac rhythm is further of two types, regular irregularity and irregular irregularity.

On the basis of pattern of regularity, any cardiac rhythm can thus be classified as:

- Regular rhythm
- Irregular rhythm
  - Regularly irregular rhythm
  - Irregularly irregular rhythm

Almost all sinus rhythms including sinus bradycardia and sinus tachycardia as well as fast rhythms such as atrial, junctional and ventricular tachycardias are regular rhythms. Examples of regularly irregular rhythms are:

- Premature beats during any rhythm
- Regular pauses during any rhythm
- Beats in pairs; bigeminal rhythm.

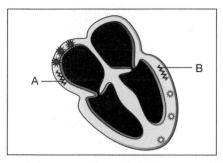

Fig. 5.6: Myocardial activation during fibrillation: (A) Atrial fibrillation; (B) Ventricular fibrillation

Fibrillation is the prototype of an irregularly irregular rhythm. Fibrillation is characterized by the functional fragmentation of the atrial or ventricular myocardium into numerous tissue islets in various stages of excitation and recovery **(Fig. 5.6)**. Myocardial depolarization is thus chaotic and ineffectual in pumping.

In atrial fibrillation, the discrete P waves of sinus rhythm are replaced by numerous, small irregularly occurring fibrillatory waves of variable morphology. These fibrillatory waves produce a ragged baseline or a straight line with minimal undulations between QRS complexes.

The RR interval is highly variable and the heart rate grossly irregular, as out of the numerous fibrillatory waves, only a few can activate the ventricles and that too at random. The QRS complexes are normal in morphology since the intraventricular conduction proceeds as usual.

Ventricular fibrillation manifests itself with rapid, irregularly occurring, small deformed deflections, grossly variable in shape, height and width. The regular waveforms of P waves, QRS complexes and T waves are distorted beyond recognition and the baseline seems to waver unevenly.

Atrioventricular Relationship

The normal cardiac activation sequence is such that the electrical impulse from the SA node first activates the atria and then travels downwards through the conducting system to activate the ventricles. We know that atrial depolarization is represented by the P wave and ventricular depolarization is represented by the QRS complex. Therefore, the P wave is followed by the QRS complex and the two are related to each other.

Imagine, a situation in which the atria are governed by the SA node while the ventricles are governed by a subsidiary pacemaker located in the AV junction or the ventricle. In that case, the atria and ventricles will beat independent of each other **(Fig. 5.7)**, and the P waves will be unrelated to the QRS complexes. This is precisely what is meant by atrioventricular dissociation (AV dissociation).

There are various electrocardiographic conditions that produce AV dissociation. The first situation is one in which a junctional/ventricular pacemaker undergoes an enhancement of automaticity and activates the ventricles at a rate faster than the rate at which the SA node activates the atria.

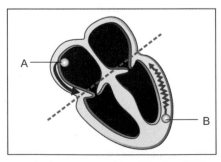

Fig. 5.7: Atrioventricular dissociation: (A) Atrial rhythm; (B) Ventricular rhythm

TABLE 5.2: Various arrhythmias causing AV dissociation

	Idiojunctional tachycardia	Idioventricular tachycardia	Complete AV block
Atrial rate	70–80 (normal)	70–80 (normal)	70–80 (normal)
Junctional rate	70–100 (slightly faster)	—	40–60 (slightly slower) or
Ventricular rate	—	70–100 (slightly faster)	20–40 (much slower)

In that case, the P waves will either be unrelated to the QRS complexes or alternatively, they will be buried in the wide QRS complexes. The RR intervals may be slightly shorter than the PP intervals (ventricular rate slightly more than atrial rate). This allows the PR interval to progressively shorten till the P wave merges into the QRS complex.

Secondly, if there is complete AV nodal block, no atrial beat is followed by or related to a ventricular beat and the P waves occur independent of the QRS complexes. However, the PP and RR intervals are constant. The relative rate of discharge of the atrial and ventricular pacemakers depends upon the condition causing AV dissociation. This is shown in **Table 5.2**.

In AV dissociation, the P wave retains its normal morphology as the atria are governed by the SA node as usual. The morphology of the QRS complex depends upon the site of the subsidiary pacemaker.

If the pacemaker is junctional, the QRS complex is normal and narrow as ventricular activation occurs through the specialized conduction system. If the pacemaker is ventricular, the QRS complex is abnormal and wide as ventricular activation then occurs through ordinary myocardium.

6

Abnormalities of the P Wave

NORMAL P WAVE

The P wave is produced by atrial depolarization. It is the sum of right and left atrial activation, the right atrium being activated first, since the pacemaker is located in it. The normal P wave meets the following criteria:

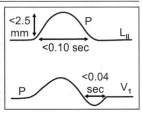

- It is upright in most leads (except aVR, V_1)
- It is constant in morphology, beat to beat
- It has a single peak and it is not notched
- It is less than 2.5 mm (0.25 mV) in height
- It is less than 2.5 mm (0.10 second) in width.

ABSENT P WAVE

The P waves are not discernible in the following conditions:
- *Atrial fibrillation:* In atrial fibrillation, P waves are replaced by numerous, small, irregularly occurring fibrillatory waves, producing a ragged baseline
- *Atrial flutter:* In atrial flutter, P waves are replaced by flutter waves (F waves) that give the baseline a corrugated or saw-toothed appearance

- *Junctional rhythm:* In a junctional rhythm, P waves may just precede, just follow or are buried in the QRS complexes due to near simultaneous activation of the ventricles anterogradely and the atria retrogradely
- *Ventricular tachycardia:* In ventricular tachycardia, P waves are difficult to identify as they lie buried in the wide QRS complexes
- *Hyperkalemia:* In hyperkalemia, P waves are reduced in amplitude or altogether absent. This is associated with tall T waves and wide QRS complexes.

INVERTED P WAVE

The P waves are normally upright in leads L_{II}, L_{III} and aVF, since the atria are activated above downwards towards the inferior leads. If activation of the atria occurs retrogradely from below upwards, the P waves in these leads are negative or inverted. Inverted P waves are thus observed in the following conditions:

- *Junctional rhythm:* In a junctional rhythm, inverted P waves may just precede or just follow the QRS complexes.
- *Bypass tract:* Inverted P waves are seen, if the atria are activated retrogradely through an accessory pathway bypassing the AV node. This is known as a bypass tract and occurs in Wolff-Parkinson-White (WPW) syndrome.

CHANGING P WAVE MORPHOLOGY

Normally, all the P waves in a given ECG strip are of identical morphology, reflecting a constant pattern of atrial activation. If impulses arise from different foci other than the SA node, the pattern of atrial activation varies from beat to beat. This produces P waves of different morphology, known as P' waves. P' waves are observed in the following rhythms:

- *Wandering pacemaker rhythm:* In this rhythm, the pace-maker, so to say, wanders from one focus to the other. The focus of origin of impulses varies from SA node to atrium to AV junction. This results in P waves of variable morphology.

- *Multifocal atrial tachycardia:* In this rhythm, impulses arise from multiple atrial foci to produce an atrial tachy-cardia or a chaotic pattern of atrial activation. Therefore, the P wave configuration changes from beat to beat.

In both the above rhythms, three kinds of P waves may be observed. Ectopic P' waves are upright, but different from sinus P waves and are atrial in origin. Retrograde P' waves are inverted and are junctional in origin. Fusion beats are P waves having a morphology in between that of a sinus P wave and an ectopic P' wave.

Interestingly, wandering pacemaker (WPM) rhythm and multifocal atrial tachycardia (MAT) only differ in terms of the heart rate. WPM rhythm occurs at a rate less than 100 beats/minute, while the rate exceeds 100 beats/minute in MAT.

TALL P WAVE

The normal P wave is less than 2.5 mm in height. It is the sum of right and left atrial activation, right preceding the left. If the right atrium is enlarged, the deflection of the right atrium is superimposed on the left atrial deflection, resulting in a tall P wave exceeding 2.5 mm in height.

Therefore, a tall P wave is representative of right atrial enlargement **(Fig. 6.1A).** Of the biphasic P wave in lead V_1, as the initial component is larger **(Fig. 6.1B).** A tall P wave is also known as P pulmonale, since it is often caused by pulmonary hypertension or P congenitale, as it may be observed in congenital heart disease.

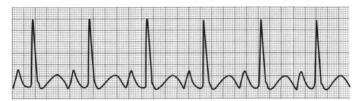

Fig. 6.1A: P. pulmonale: Tall and peaked P wave

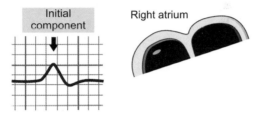

Fig. 6.1B: P wave in V₁: Large initial component

BROAD P WAVE

The normal P wave is less than 2.5 mm or 0.10 second in width. It is the sum of right and left atrial activation, right preceding the left. If the left atrium is enlarged, the deflection of the left atrium is further delayed after the right atrial deflection, resulting in a broad P wave exceeding 2.5 mm in width. Also, a notch appears on the P wave, between its right and left atrial components.

Therefore, a broad and notched P wave is representative of left atrial enlargement **(Fig. 6.2A)**. Of the biphasic P wave in lead V_1, the terminal component is larger **(Fig. 6.2B)**. A broad and notched P wave is also known as P mitrale, since it is often associated with mitral valve disease.

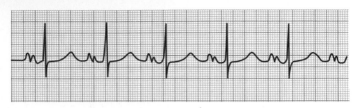

Fig. 6.2A: P mitrale: Broad and notched P wave

Left atrium

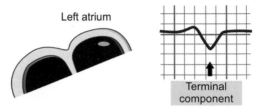

Terminal component

Fig. 6.2B: P wave in V₁: Large terminal component

TABLE 6.1: Various causes of atrial enlargement

	Left atrial enlargement	Right atrial enlargement
Intracardiac shunt	Ventricular septal defect (VSD)	Atrial septal defect (ASD)
AV valve disease	Mitral stenosis Mitral regurgitation	Tricuspid stenosis Tricuspid regurgitation
Outflow obstruction	Aortic stenosis	Pulmonary stenosis
Hypertension	Systemic hypertension	Pulmonary hypertension
Myocardial disease	Cardiomyopathy	Cor pulmonale

The common causes of atrial enlargement have been enumerated in **Table 6.1** and the abnormalities of P wave morphology in right atrial and left atrial enlargement are illustrated in **Figure 6.3.**

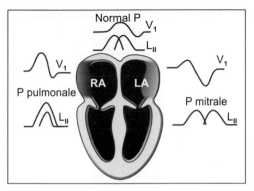

Fig. 6.3: P wave abnormalities in right and left atrial enlargement

Abnormalities of QRS Complex

NORMAL QRS COMPLEX

The QRS complex is produced by ventricular depolarization. It is the sum of synchronized activation of the right and left ventricles. The normal QRS complex meets the following criteria:

- R wave voltage is at least 5 mm in the limb leads and at least 10 mm in the precordial leads
- There is normally no variation in the QRS voltage of consecutive beats in a particular lead
- The normal QRS axis ranges from –30° to +90° on the hexaxial reference system
- R wave magnitude increases gradually from lead V_1 to lead V_6 representing transition from right ventricular to left ventricular QRS complexes
- Physiological q waves are seen in leads L_I, aVL. They are less than 25 percent of the ensuing R wave in size and less than 0.04 second in duration
- R wave voltage does not exceed 4 mm in lead V_1 and is not more than 25 mm in lead V_5 and V_6

- The normal S wave is larger than the r wave in lead V_1 and smaller than the R wave in lead V_6. It does not exceed a depth of 7 mm in lead V_6
- The width of the normal QRS complex does not exceed 0.08 second or 2 small squares.

LOW VOLTAGE QRS COMPLEX

The voltage of the R wave in the QRS complex is normally at least 5 mm in the limb leads and at least 10 mm in the precordial leads. If the voltage of the tallest R wave in the limb leads is less than 5 mm and that in the precordial leads is less than 10 mm, the electrocardiogram obtained is called, a low voltage graph.

The magnitude of the R wave depends upon the quantum of electrical forces that are generated by the left ventricle as well as on the extent to which these electrical forces are transmitted to the recording electrode.

Therefore, a low voltage graph may be obtained, if the myocardium is diseased, or if an abnormal substance or tissue intervenes between the epicardial surface of the heart and the recording electrode **(Fig. 7.1).**

Accordingly, the causes of a low voltage ECG graph can be classified as follows:

- *Due to low voltage generation*
    - ⟼ Hypothyroidism
    - ⟼ Hypopituitarism
    - ⟼ Constrictive pericarditis

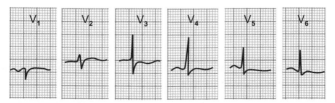

Fig. 7.1: Hypothyroidism: Low voltage graph; T wave inversion

➡ Diffuse myocardial disease
➡ Incorrect standardization.
- *Due to intervening substance/tissue*
  ➡ Adipose tissue in obesity
  ➡ Muscle in thick chest wall
  ➡ Fluid in pericardial effusion
  ➡ Air in pulmonary emphysema.

The cause of a low QRS voltage graph can be assessed by analysis of these parameters:
- The heart rate
- The clinical profile
- The QRS-T shape.

One vital technical point; before the diagnosis of low QRS voltages is made, it must be ensured that the ECG machine has been properly standardized. Accurate standardization means that a one millivolt current produces a 10 mm tall deflection.

ALTERNATING QRS VOLTAGE

Normally, in a given lead, the voltage of all the QRS complexes is the same. This is because all beats originate from one pacemaker and the voltage has no relation to respiration or any other periodic extracardiac phenomenon.

If the voltage of QRS complexes alternates between high and low in successive beats, the condition is known as electrical alternans **(Fig. 7.2).** Total electrical alternans refers to a condition wherein, the voltage of the P wave, T wave and QRS complex are all variable from beat-to-beat.

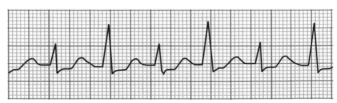

Fig. 7.2: Electrical alternans: Varying voltage of the QRS complex

Electrical alternans is caused either by a positional oscillation of the heart within a fluid-filled pericardial sac or a beat-to-beat variation in the aberrancy of intraventricular conduction. Accordingly, the causes of electrical alternans are:

- Moderate to severe pericardial effusion
  - ⟶ Malignant
  - ⟶ Tubercular
  - ⟶ Postsurgical.
- Serious organic heart disease
  - ⟶ Ischemic cardiomyopathy
  - ⟶ Diffuse myocarditis.

Total electrical alternans is highly suggestive of moderate to severe pericardial effusion with cardiac tamponade or impending tamponade. Electrical alternans of the QRS complex is often clinically associated with cardiomegaly, gallop rhythm and signs of left ventricular decompensation.

ABNORMAL QRS AXIS

The dominant direction of the net electrical forces constitutes the electrical axis of the QRS complex. Normally, these forces are so directed that the QRS axis is in the range of –30° to +90° on the hexaxial reference system.

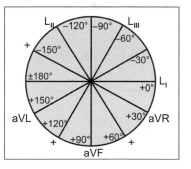

In other words, the QRS axis falls in the right lower quadrant of the hexaxial system. This means that the main QRS deflection in both leads L_I as well as aVF is upright. This is also known as the "2 thumbs-up sign".

TABLE 7.1: QRS electrical axis from the hexaxial system

QRS axis	Range in degrees
Normal axis	− 30° to +90°
Left axis deviation	− 30° to −90°
Right axis deviation	+ 90° to +180°
Indeterminate axis	− 90° to −180°

Abnormalities of the QRS axis include:
- Right axis deviation
- Left axis deviation
- Indeterminate axis.

On a scale of 360 degrees (0° to +180° and 0° to –180°), the entire hexaxial system is used to qualify the QRS axis as shown in **Table 7.1.**

We have seen that although the QRS axis is generally calculated mathematically, we can know the quadrant into which the axis falls by scanning the direction of the main deflection (positive or negative) in leads L_I and aVF. Accordingly, the QRS axis can be classified as in **Table 7.2.**

Causes of deviation of the QRS axis are:
- *Right axis deviation*
  ➠ Thin tall built
  ➠ Right ventricular hypertrophy
  ➠ Left posterior hemiblock
  ➠ Anterolateral infarction
  ➠ Chronic lung disease

TABLE 7.2: QRS electrical axis from the leads L_I and aVF

Main deflection in L_I	aVF	QRS quadrant	QRS axis
+ve	+ve	Right lower	0° to +90°
+ve	−ve	Right upper	0° to −90°
−ve	+ve	Left lower	+90° to +180°
−ve	−ve	Left upper	−90° to −180°

⮕ Pulmonary embolism

⮕ Ostium secundum atrial septal defect (ASD).

- *Left axis deviation*
  ⮕ Obese stocky built
  ⮕ Left ventricular hypertrophy
  ⮕ Left anterior hemiblock
  ⮕ Inferior wall infarction
  ⮕ Wolff-Parkinson-White (WPW) syndrome
  ⮕ Ostium primum ASD
  ⮕ Ventricular tachycardia.
- *Indeterminate (North-West) axis*
  ⮕ Severe right ventricular hypertrophy
  ⮕ Aneurysm of left ventricular apex.

Deviation of the QRS axis can occur due to various physiological as well as pathological causes. Age and body habitus are important determinants of the QRS axis.

Minor right axis deviation can occur in thin, lean children and adolescents. Minor left axis deviation is normal in obese adults and with abdominal distension due to pregnancy or ascites.

FASCICULAR BLOCK OR HEMIBLOCK

The intraventricular conducting system consists of a bundle of His, which divides into right and left bundle branches. The left bundle branch further divides into an anterior fascicle and a posterior fascicle.

A block in conduction, down one of the fascicles results in abnormal left ventricular activation known as hemiblock. Thus, we have left anterior hemiblock and left posterior hemiblock. A hemiblock produces significant deviation of the QRS axis.

In left anterior hemiblock, there is qR pattern in lead L_I and rS pattern in lead aVF or left axis deviation **(Fig. 7.3A).**

In left posterior hemiblock, there is rS pattern in lead L₁ and qR pattern in lead aVF or right axis deviation **(Fig. 7.3B)**.

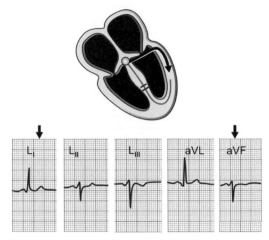

Fig. 7.3A: Left axis deviation: Left anterior fascicular block

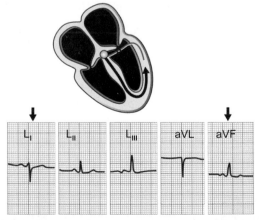

Fig. 7.3B: Right axis deviation: Left posterior fascicular block

Left anterior hemiblock (LAHB) may be observed in:

- Hypertension with LV hypertrophy
- Calcification from aortic valve
- Chronic coronary insufficiency
- Chronic dilated cardiomyopathy
- Fibrocalcerous degeneration.

LAHB is more common and often occurs alone. This is because the anterior fascicle is long, thin, has a single blood supply and commonly gets involved in diseases affecting the septum and aortic valve.

Left posterior hemiblock (LPHB) may be observed in:

- Inferior wall infarction
- Right bundle branch block.

LPHB is less common and rarely occurs alone. This is because the posterior fascicle is short, thick, has a dual blood supply and is uncommonly involved in diseases affecting the septum and aortic valve.

NONPROGRESSION OF R WAVE

Normally, as we move across the precordial leads from lead V_1 to lead V_6, there is a progressive increase in R wave voltage. This is because the right ventricular leads V_1, V_2 record rS complexes while the left ventricular leads V_5, V_6 record qR complexes.

The change from rS pattern to qR pattern generally occurs in lead V_3 or V_4, which is known as the transition zone. In the transition zone, the QRS complex is isoelectric with the R wave height and S wave depth being almost equal **(Fig. 7.4A)**.

The vector can rotate in the horizontal plane with the transitional QRS moving towards the patient's right or left. When it moves to the right (into leads V_1, V_2), this is rightward rotation. When it moves to the left (into leads V_5, V_6), this is leftward rotation. As a rule, the vector shifts towards ventricular hypertrophy and away from myocardial infarction. Failure of the R wave voltage to increase progressively from lead V_1 to lead V_6 is referred to as nonprogression of the R wave (**Fig. 7.4B**) or leftward rotation.

Causes of nonprogression of the R wave are:

- Chronic lung disease
- Old anteroseptal infarction
- Diffuse myocardial disease
- Left ventricular hypertrophy
- Left bundle branch block.

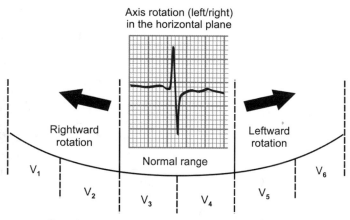

Fig. 7.4A: Rotation of the vector and shift of transition zone

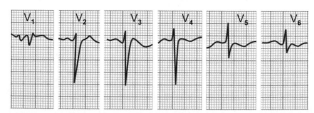

Fig. 7.4B: Nonprogression of R wave in the precordial leads

Nonprogression of the R wave in precordial leads can occur due to a variety of causes. Knowledge of this fact can avoid the overdiagnosis of ominous conditions like old myocardial infarction.

Even improper placement of chest electrodes can produce this striking abnormality, particularly in the situation of a medical emergency.

ABNORMAL Q WAVES

The Q waves are not visible in all ECG leads. Rather, they are normally visible in selected leads where they represent initial septal activation in a direction opposite to activation of the main left ventricular mass.

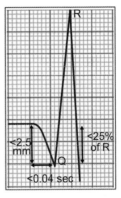

Physiological Q waves are observed in:

- Leads L_I, aVL, with horizontal heart
- Leads L_{III}, aVF with a vertical heart.

Criteria for physiological Q waves are:

- They do not exceed 0.04 second in duration
- They do not exceed one-fourth of R wave height.

Pathological Q waves are most commonly due to necrosis of heart muscle or myocardial infarction. This is a result of occlusion of a coronary artery by a thrombus **(Fig. 7.5).** Why pathological Q waves appear in myocardial infarction needs to be understood. Infarcted (necrotic) myocardial tissue is electrically inert and does not get depolarized. If an electrode is placed over this "electrical hole" or "void", it records depolarization of the opposite ventricular wall from the endocardium to the epicardium.

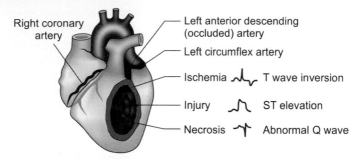

Fig. 7.5: Zones of myocardial infarction and their ECG effects

Since, this direction of depolarization is away from the electrode, the recorded deflection is negative and is called the Q wave **(Fig. 7.6).** The Q wave may be followed by a small r wave or there may be an entirely negative deflection, (QS complex).

Pathological Q waves meet the following criteria:
- More than or equal to 0.04 second in duration
- More than one-fourth of R wave amplitude
- Present in several leads and not an isolated lead
- Isolated q waves in lead L_{III} may disappear on deep inspiration.

Pathological Q waves occur commonly, but not always due to myocardial infarction. Severe reversible myocardial ischemia as in severe angina, hypoxia, hypothermia or hypoglycemia may cause transient appearance of Q waves.

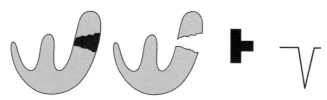

Fig. 7.6: Electrode placed over transmural infarct records negative deflection: The "electrical hole" effect

TABLE 7.3: Area of infarction determined from Q wave location

Location of Q wave	Area of infarction
V_1, V_2	Septal
V_3, V_4	Anterior
V_5, V_6, L_I, aVL	Lateral
V_{1-4}	Anteroseptal
V_{3-6}, L_I, aVL	Anterolateral
V_{1-6}, L_I, aVL	Extensive anterior
L_I, aVL	High lateral
L_{II}, L_{III}, aVF	Inferior

Absence of Q waves does not rule out the possibility of myocardial infarction. Q waves may be absent in the following types of infarction—small infarction, right ventricular infarction, posterior wall infarction, atrial infarction and fresh infarction with delayed ECG changes. The location of Q waves can help to localize the area of infarction as tabulated in **Table 7.3**.

ABNORMALLY TALL R WAVES

The r wave voltage in lead V_1 represents rightward forces while the R wave height in lead V_6 represents left ventricular forces. Normally, the R wave amplitude does not exceed 4 mm in lead V_1 and does not exceed 25 mm in lead V_6. Also, the R wave height is less than S wave depth (R/S ratio less than 1) in lead V_1 and more than the S wave depth (R/S ratio more than 1) in lead V_6.

A R wave greater than 4 mm in lead V_1 is considered tall. Causes of tall R waves in lead V_1 are:
- Right ventricular hypertrophy
- Right bundle branch block
- Persistent juvenile pattern

- True posterior wall infarction
- Mirror-image dextrocardia
- Pre-excitation (WPW syndrome)
- Acute pulmonary embolism.

A, R wave greater than 25 mm in lead V_6 is considered tall. Causes of tall R waves in lead V_6 are:

- Left ventricular hypertrophy
- Left bundle branch block.

Right Ventricular Hypertrophy (RVH)

The QRS complex represents ventricular depolarization. Therefore, the tall R wave in lead V_1 in right ventricular hypertrophy reflects the increased electrical forces generated by the thickened right ventricular myocardium.

The voltage criteria of RVH are:

- R wave in V_1 more than 4 mm
- R/S ratio in V_1 more than 1
- S wave in V_6 more than 7 mm
- R in V_1 + S in V_6 more than 10 mm.

Besides voltage criteria, other features of RVH are:

- Right axis deviation of the QRS complex
- Right atrial enlargement: P pulmonale
- S-T segment depression and T wave inversion in leads V_1 and V_2: The RV strain pattern **(Fig. 7.7).**

The causes of RVH can be classified into causes of pulmonary hypertension and those of pulmonary stenosis. These are:

- *Pulmonary hypertension*
  - ➡ Congenital heart disease (intracardiac shunt)
  - ➡ Mitral valve disease (stenosis or regurgitation)
  - ➡ Chronic pulmonary disease (cor pulmonale)
  - ➡ Primary pulmonary hypertension (idiopathic).

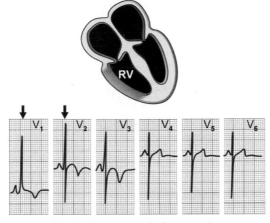

Fig. 7.7: Right ventricular hypertrophy:
Tall R wave in V₁ to V₃; rS pattern in V₄ to V₆

- *Pulmonary stenosis (PS)*
  - ➠ Isolated congenital PS
  - ➠ PS of Fallot's tetralogy.

In pulmonary hypertension, there is increased resistance to blood flow in the pulmonary vasculature. In pulmonary stenosis, there is obstruction to right ventricular outflow at the level of pulmonary valve.

Right ventricular hypertrophy is common, but by no means, the only cause of tall R waves in lead V_1. It needs to be differentiated from the following conditions that also produce tall R waves in lead V_1.

Persistent Juvenile Pattern

The right ventricle is the dominant ventricle in childhood. Sometimes, the juvenile pattern of right ventricular dominance persists into adulthood to cause a dominantly upright deflection in lead V_1.

Right Bundle Branch Block (RBBB)

In RBBB, the dominant deflection in lead V_1 is upright. But close analysis of the QRS complex reveals a wide deflection (>0.12 second in width) with a triphasic contour that produces a M-pattern or RsR' configuration.

Posterior Wall Infarction

None of the electrocardiographic leads are oriented towards the posterior wall of the heart. Therefore, the diagnosis of posterior wall infarction is made from the inverse of classical changes of infarction in lead V_1.

These include a tall R wave and an upright T wave, which are the reverse of a deep Q wave and an inverted T wave. Note that posterior wall infarction is the only cause of tall R wave in V_1, in which the T wave is also tall and upright.

Mirror-image Dextrocardia

In mirror-image dextrocardia, since the heart lies in the right side of the chest and lead V_1 overlies the left ventricle, the R wave is tallest in lead V_1 and diminishes towards lead V_6.

The WPW Syndrome

The WPW syndrome or pre-excitation syndrome is often associated with upright QRS complexes in right precordial leads V_1, V_2. Other electrocardiographic features of WPW syndrome include a short P-R interval and a delta wave deforming the normally smooth ascending limb of the R wave.

Left Ventricular Hypertrophy (LVH)

The QRS complex represents ventricular depolarization. Therefore, the tall R wave in lead V_5 in left ventricular hypertrophy reflects the increased electrical forces generated by the thickened left ventricular myocardium.

The voltage criteria of LVH are:

- S in V_1 + R in (V_5 or V_6)   >35 mm (Sokolow)
- R in V_4–V_6 >25 mm; R in aVL   >11 mm (Framingham)
- S in V_3 + R in aVL   >28 mm in men (Cornell)

Besides voltage criteria, other features of LVH are:

- Left axis deviation of the QRS complex
- Left atrial enlargement: P mitrale
- ST segment depression and T wave inversion in leads V_5 and V_6: LV strain pattern **(Fig. 7.8).**

The causes of LVH can be classified into causes of systolic LV overload and those of diastolic LV overload. These are:

- *Systolic LV overload*
  - ⟹ Systemic hypertension
  - ⟹ Aortic stenosis
    - ◊ Valvular
    - ◊ Subvalvular

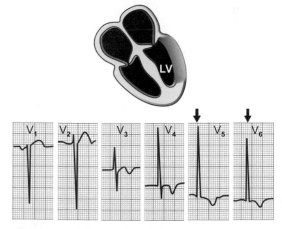

Fig. 7.8: Left ventricular hypertrophy: Tall R wave in V_5, V_6; deep S wave in V_1, V_2

➡ Coarctation of aorta
➡ Hypertrophic cardiomyopathy.
• *Diastolic LV overload*
➡ Aortic regurgitation
➡ Mitral incompetence
➡ Ventricular septal defect
➡ Patent ductus arteriosus.

In systolic overload, there is increased resistance to outflow of arterial blood from the left ventricle. In diastolic overload, there is an increased inflow of venous blood to the left ventricle.

Left ventricular hypertrophy is common but by no means, the only cause of tall R wave in V_6. It needs to be differentiated from other conditions that cause tall R wave.

• *Voltage criteria alone:* The voltage criteria of LVH can be fulfilled by high cardiac output states such as anemia, thyrotoxicosis and beri-beri. Similarly, strenuous exercisers, conditioned athletes and marathon runners can have tall R waves in lead V_6.

However, in these conditions, the voltage criteria are not accompanied by other ECG features of LVH such as left axis deviation, strain pattern or P mitrale. Moreover, their clinical evaluation is unremarkable. Therefore, one must be careful before diagnosing left ventricular hypertrophy by voltage criteria alone.

• *Left bundle branch block (LBBB):* In LBBB, the QRS deflection in lead V_6 is tall. But close analysis of the QRS complex reveals a wide deflection (> 0.12 second in width) with a triphasic contour that produces a M-pattern or RsR' configuration.

• *Left ventricular diastolic overload:* In true left ventricular hypertrophy or systolic overload, the tall R wave without a preceding Q wave is classically associated with depression of the ST segment and inversion of the T wave, the so called left ventricular strain pattern.

Left ventricular diastolic overload can be differentiated from systolic overload by certain subtle differences. In diastolic overload, the tall R wave is preceded by a deep narrow Q wave and associated with a tall and upright T wave.

ABNORMALLY DEEP S WAVES

The S wave in lead V_1 represents left ventricular activation while in lead V_6 it represents right ventricular activation. Normally, the S wave depth in lead V_1 is greater than the r wave height. Also, the s wave is much smaller than the R wave in lead V_6 and does not exceed 7 mm in depth.

In lead V_1, if the s wave is smaller than the R wave and the R/S ratio is greater than 1, it indicates right ventricular dominance or hypertrophy **(Fig. 7.7).** If the sum of S wave voltage in lead V_1 and R wave voltage in lead V_6 exceeds 35 mm, it indicates left ventricular hypertrophy **(Fig. 7.8).**

It is interesting to note that the lead V_1 provides a wealth of information concerning hypertrophy of the cardiac chambers.

- LV hypertrophy : Deep S wave, small r wave
- RV hypertrophy : Tall R wave small s wave
- LA enlargement : Large terminal P component
- RA enlargement : Large initial P component.

ABNORMALLY WIDE QRS COMPLEXES

The QRS complex represents depolarization of the entire ventricular myocardium. Since the right and left ventricles are depolarized in a synchronous fashion, the normal QRS width does not exceed 0.04–0.08 second (1 to 2 small squares) on the horizontal or time axis.

If the QRS complex is wider than 0.08 second, it means that either the two ventricles are activated asynchronously or ventricular conduction is slow. Causes of wide QRS complexes are:

- Bundle branch block
  - ➠ Right bundle branch block
  - ➠ Left bundle branch block.
- Intraventricular conduction defect
  - ➠ Antiarrhythmic drugs, e.g. amiodarone
  - ➠ Electrolyte imbalance, e.g. hyperkalemia
  - ➠ Myocardial disease, e.g. myocarditis.
- Ventricular preexcitation
  - ➠ WPW syndrome
  - ➠ LGL syndrome.
- Wide QRS arrhythmias
  - ➠ Supraventricular tachycardia with aberrant ventricular conduction.

The causes of wide QRS complexes can also be classified according to the width of the complexes:

- QRS width 0.09–0.10 second
  - ➠ Left anterior or posterior hemiblock
  - ➠ Partial intraventricular conduction defect
- QRS width 0.11–0.12 second
  - ➠ Incomplete bundle branch block
  - ➠ Intraventricular conduction defect
  - ➠ Ventricular preexcitation syndrome.
- QRS width > 0.12 second
  - ➠ Bundle branch block
  - ➠ Wide QRS arrhythmias.

Bundle Branch Block

Bundle branch block denotes a delay or block of conduction down one of the two branches of the bundle of His. Accordingly, we can have right bundle branch block (RBBB) or left bundle branch block (LBBB). Bundle branch block produces widening of the QRS complex because of delayed activation of one of the ventricles, right ventricle in RBBB and left ventricle in LBBB. Depolarization of the blocked ventricle occurs slowly through the myocardium and not by the specialized conduction system.

An incomplete bundle branch block results in a QRS width of 0.11–0.12 second while in a complete block, the QRS width exceeds 0.12 second. Bundle branch block produces a RSR' pattern or M-shaped QRS deflection with two peaks. The QRS complexes of the ventricles are "out of sync" with each other and produce two R waves in sequential order.

In RBBB, the RSR' pattern is observed in lead V_1, the R' wave representing delayed right ventricular activation **(Fig. 7.9)**. In LBBB, the M-shaped pattern is observed in lead V_6, the notched R wave representing delayed left ventricular activation **(Fig. 7.10)**. The RSR' complex is followed by ST segment depression and T wave inversion which together constitute secondary ST-T changes of bundle branch block.

Bundle branch block often indicates organic heart disease, more so LBBB. On the other hand, RBBB is occasionally observed in normal individuals. Causes of left bundle branch block are:

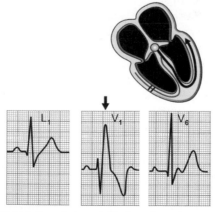

Fig. 7.9: Right bundle branch block: M-shaped complex in V_1; Slurred S wave in L_1, V_6

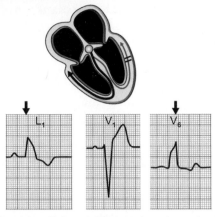

Fig. 7.10: Left bundle branch block: M-shaped complex in L_1, V_6; Wide QS complex in V_1 to V_4

- Myocardial infarction (recent or healed)
- Systemic hypertension (long-standing)
- Aortic valve disease (calcific stenosis)
- Cardiomyopathy (or acute myocarditis)
- Fibrocalcerous disease (degenerative)
- Cardiac trauma (accidental or surgical).

Causes of right bundle branch block, besides those mentioned above are:

- Atrial septal defect
  ⇒ Ostium secundum: Incomplete RBBB
  ⇒ Ostium primum: RBBB + LAHB
- Acute pulmonary embolism
- Arrhythmogenic RV dysplasia
- Chronic pulmonary disease.

RBBB does not distort the QRS complex, but only adds a terminal deflection which is the R' wave in leads V_1, V_2 and slurred S wave in leads L_1, V_6. On the other hand, LBBB totally distorts the QRS complex. Therefore, it is possible to diagnose myocardial infarction in the presence of RBBB, but difficult in the presence of LBBB. Criteria for the diagnosis of myocardial infarction in the presence of LBBB are:

- Presence of Q wave in L_1, aVL, V_5, V_6
- Terminal S wave in the leads V_5, V_6
- Upright T wave concordant with QRS
- ST drift > 5 mm discordant with QRS.

Brugada Syndrome

The Brugada syndrome also produces a rSR' pattern in lead V_1 with saddle-back shaped ST elevation and T wave inversion, which superficially resembles a RBBB pattern **(Fig. 7.11)**. But unlike in RBBB, the rSR' is not more than 0.12 second wide and there are no slurred S waves in leads L_1 and V_6.

The Brugada syndrome is a rare congenital disorder of sodium transport, across ion channels in the right ventricle. Patients with this condition are prone to develop episodic syncope due to ventricular tachycardia or even cardiac arrest due to ventricular fibrillation. The genetic defect underlying Brugada syndrome may exist in several family members (autosomal dominant inheritance) and forms the basis of familial malignant ventricular arrhythmias requiring an implantable cardioverter defibrillator (ICD).

Brugada syndrome belongs to a group of congenital channelopathies responsible for 5–10% of cases of

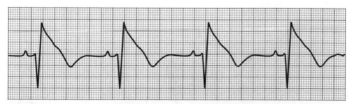

Fig. 7.11: Brugada syndrome: rSR' pattern in lead V_1; Normal rSR' duration; Elevated ST segment; Inverted T wave

sudden cardiac death (SCD). Other channelopathies are long QT syndrome (LQTS) and catecholaminergic ventricular tachycardia (CVT).

Arrhythmogenic RV Dysplasia

Arrhythmogenic right ventricular dysplasia (ARVD) produces incomplete right bundle branch block (RBBB) pattern with a postdepolarization epsilon wave at the end of the QRS complex, best seen in lead V_1. There is also T wave inversion in the right precordial leads V_1–V_4.

Echocardiography reveals a mildly dilated right ventricle with akinetic regions due to substitution of portions of the right ventricular musculature with fibrotic adipose tissue. A definitive diagnosis of ARVD comes from magnetic resonance imaging (MRI). Electrophysiology study demonstrates inducible polymorphic ventricular tachycardia. These patients merit lifelong arrhythmia prophylaxis with a beta-blocker or an implantable cardioverter defibrillator (ICD).

Acute Pulmonary Embolism

Pulmonary embolism causing acute cor pulmonale, is a prominent cause of acute onset right bundle branch block. Various ECG features of acute pulmonary embolism are:

- Sinus tachycardia (invariable)
- Atrial fibrillation (occasional)
- Incomplete/complete RBBB
- Dominant R wave in V_1
- T wave inversion V_1–V_3
- Right ward QRS axis
- Tall P wave (P pulmonale)
- A typical $S_1Q_3T_3$ pattern
  S in L_I, Q in L_{III}, T in L_{III}

Chronic Pulmonary Disease

Chronic obstructive pulmonary disease (COPD) with cor pulmonale can also cause right bundle branch block (RBBB). Various ECG features of COPD are:

- Low voltage QRS complexes
- Right ventricular hypertrophy
- Right atrial enlargement
- Rightward QRS axis deviation
- Atrial fibrillation (AF) or even multifocal atrial tachycardia.

Intraventricular Conduction Defect

An intraventricular conduction defect (IVCD) refers to a delay or block in conduction in the Purkinje system, distal to the bundle branches. It produces widening of the QRS complex since the ventricular muscle has to be activated through ordinary myocardium, instead of the specialized conduction tissue. As we have seen earlier, an IVCD may occur due to antiarrhythmic drugs, electrolyte imbalance or primary myocardial disease.

Antiarrhythmic drugs such as amiodarone, widen the QRS complex. A widening beyond 25 percent of the baseline value is an indication of drug toxicity.

Other ECG effects of antiarrhythmic drugs are:

- ST depression and T inversion
- Prolongation of QT interval
- Prominence of U wave **(Fig. 7.12)**.

Hyperkalemia, if severe (serum K^+ more than 9 mEq/L), results in a QRS complex that is wide and bizarre.

Other ECG features of hyperkalemia are:

- Tall, peaked T waves
- Short QT interval
- Flat P waves **(Fig. 7.13)**.

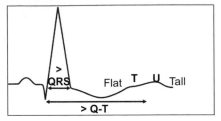

Fig. 7.12: Effects of amiodarone

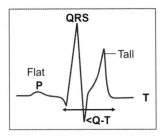

Fig. 7.13: Effects of hyperkalemia

Disease processes primarily affecting the myocardium such as cardiomyopathy or myocarditis produce total distortion and widening of the QRS complex. Low voltages of these complexes may cause poor progression of R wave in precordial leads.

Ventricular Preexcitation (WPW Syndrome)

The WPW syndrome is an entity in which an accessory pathway or bypass tract called the bundle of Kent connects the atrial to the ventricular myocardium, without passing through the AV node.

Conduction of impulses down this tract results in premature ventricular activation also called preexcitation, since the AV nodal delay is bypassed. Conduction of an impulse through

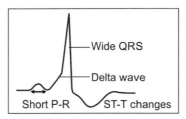

Fig. 7.14: WPW syndrome

the usual conduction system follows the preexcitation. The WPW syndrome is associated with the following ECG features:

- *Wide QRS complex*: The QRS complex is wide, since it is the sum of ventricular preexcitation by the accessory pathway and normal ventricular activation
- *Delta wave:* Preexcitation of the ventricle produces a slur on the ascending limb of R wave, termed the delta wave
- *Short PR interval:* The PR interval is short because ventricular depolarization begins early after the P wave, having bypassed the AV nodal delay
- *ST-T changes:* ST segment depression and T wave inversion are secondary to the abnormality of the QRS complex **(Fig. 7.14)**.

The clinical significance of WPW syndrome lies in the fact that it predisposes an individual to arrhythmias, particularly paroxysmal atrial tachycardia, atrial fibrillation and even ventricular tachycardia. WPW syndrome is a masquerader of several cardiac conditions. These are:

- Delta wave appearing separate from the R wave mimics bundle branch block
- Dominant R wave in lead V_1 resembles pattern of right ventricular hypertrophy
- Negative delta waves with ST-T changes give the impression of myocardial infarction
- Antidromic AV reentrant tachycardia conducted antero-gradely through the accessory pathway may be mistaken for ventricular tachycardia.

CHAPTER

8

Abnormalities of the T Wave

NORMAL T WAVE

The T wave is produced by the rapid phase of ventricular repolarization and follows the QRS complex. The normal T wave fulfills the following criteria:

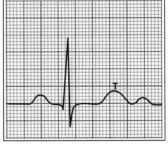

- It is upright in most leads (except aVR, L_{III}, V_1)
- It is taller in V_6 than in lead V_1 and taller in L_I than in lead L_{III}
- It does not exceed 5 mm in height in the limb leads and 10 mm in precordial leads.

INVERTED T WAVE

The T wave is considered to be the most variable component of the ECG graph. Therefore, change in polarity of the T wave or T wave inversion is one of the most common and nonspecific ECG abnormalities.

The significance of flattening or reduction in height of the T wave is similar to that of T wave inversion. Since inversion of the T wave is often associated with depression of the ST segment, together they are referred to as ST-T changes.

As the T wave is an unstable deflection, it is not surprising that T wave inversion can be caused by a wide variety of etiological factors. The causes of T wave inversion can be classified as follows:

NONSPECIFIC CAUSES

- *Physiological states*
  - ⇒ Heavy meals
  - ⇒ Smoking
  - ⇒ Anxiety
  - ⇒ Tachycardia
  - ⇒ Hyperventilation.
- *Extracardiac disorders*
  - ⇒ Systemic, e.g. hemorrhage, shock
  - ⇒ Cranial, e.g. cerebrovascular accident
  - ⇒ Abdominal, e.g. pancreatitis, cholecystitis
  - ⇒ Respiratory, e.g. pulmonary embolism
  - ⇒ Endocrine, e.g. hypothyroidism.

Specific Causes

- *Primary abnormality*
  - ⇒ Pharmacological, e.g. digitalis, quinidine
  - ⇒ Metabolic, e.g. hypokalemia, hypothermia
  - ⇒ Myocardial, e.g. cardiomyopathy, myocarditis
  - ⇒ Pericardial, e.g. pericarditis, pericardial effusion
  - ⇒ Ischemic, e.g. coronary insufficiency, infarction.
- *Secondary abnormality*
  - ⇒ Ventricular hypertrophy
  - ⇒ Bundle branch block
  - ⇒ WPW syndrome.

T wave inversion lacks specificity as a diagnostic indicator. Since inversion of the T wave can be caused by certain physiological states and noncardiac diseases, it highlights the importance of viewing T inversion in the light of clinical data.

One should be careful before diagnosing myocardial ischemia only by ECG criteria. T wave inversion should be interpreted carefully in the presence of upper abdominal and respiratory diseases, when the clinical picture may be confused with that of heart disease.

A cerebrovascular accident such as cerebral thrombosis or intracranial bleed may be associated with T wave inversion for which there are several reasons. One, there may be concomitant coronary artery disease due to common atherosclerotic risk factors. Two, the neurogenic stress response to stroke may cause acute hypertension and coronary vasoconstriction. Three, a left ventricular mural thrombus in an aneurysm may be the source of cerebral embolism.

Cardiovascular drugs like digitalis and amiodarone can cause T wave inversion and downsloping ST segment depression. With digitalis therapy, the ST segment and T wave resemble the mirror-image of the correction tick ($\sqrt{}$) **(Fig. 8.1A)**.

When these changes are confined to leads V_5, V_6, they indicate digitalis administration. Changes occurring in most leads are suggestive of digitalis intoxication.

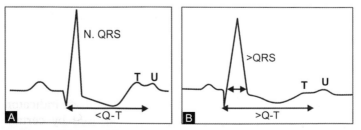

Fig. 8.1: (A) Effects of digitalis; (B) Effects of amiodarone

Antiarrhythmic drugs also causes T wave inversion and ST segment depression but unlike digitalis, they also widen the QRS complex and prolong the QT interval **(Fig. 8.1B)**.

Hypokalemia is an important cause of T wave change. The T wave is either reduced in amplitude, flattened or inverted. This is associated with prominence of the U wave that follows the T wave **(Fig. 8.2A)**. A low T wave followed by a prominent U wave produces a 'camel-hump' effect while a flat T with a prominent U falsely suggests prolongation of the QT interval **(Fig. 8.2B)**.

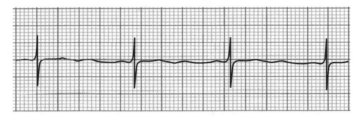

Fig. 8.2A: Effect of hypokalemia on the T wave

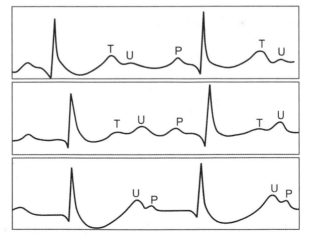

Fig. 8.2B: Effects of progressively increasing hypokalemia

Causes of hypokalemia include dietary deficiency of potassium, gastrointestinal losses in the form of vomiting and diarrhea as well as diuretic and steroid therapy. The importance of hypokalemia in cardiac patients on diuretic treatment lies in the fact that hypokalemia can precipitate digitalis toxicity and initiate ventricular tachyarrhythmias such as torsades de pointes.

Clinical features of hypokalemia are fatigue, leg cramps and neuromuscular paralysis. Treatment of hypokalemia is potassium administration, either dietary or pharmacological and correction of the underlying cause.

Primary diseases of the myocardium such as cardiomyopathy and acute myocarditis produce T wave inversion and ST segment depression. These changes are often associated with wide QRS complexes due to intraventricular conduction defect.

During the acute stage of pericarditis, the ST segment is elevated and the T wave is upright. Once the ST segment has returned to the baseline, the T wave undergoes inversion that may persist for a long time.

In pericardial effusion, T wave inversion is associated with low voltage QRS complexes. A similar pattern is observed in hypothyroidism (myxedema) with the difference that while pericardial effusion causes tachycardia, hypothyroidism is accompanied by bradycardia.

Clinically speaking, coronary artery disease with myocardial ischemia or infarction is the most important cause of T wave inversion. Acute coronary insufficiency produces coving (convexity) of the ST segment and T wave inversion **(Fig. 8.3)**. In non-Q myocardial infarction, a similar pattern is observed.

The two conditions can be differentiated by the fact that in acute coronary insufficiency, the chest pain is of short duration, cardiac enzyme titers (CPK, SGOT) are normal and

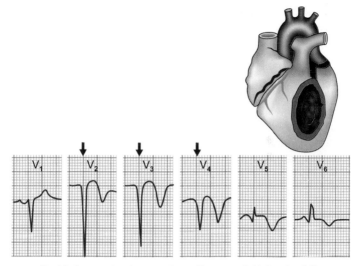

Fig. 8.3: Acute extensive anterior wall myocardial infarction fully
evolved phase: QS in V$_1$ to V$_4$; qR in V$_5$ to V$_6$

the ECG changes rapidly revert to normal with treatment. In non-Q myocardial infarction, there is history of prolonged chest pain, blood levels of cardiac enzymes are raised and the ECG changes persist for a longer period.

In the fully evolved phase of Q-wave myocardial infarction, T wave inversion is associated with elevation (convex upwards) of the ST segment **(Fig. 8.3)**. This is in contrast to the T wave inversion observed in pericarditis, which occurs after the elevated (concave upwards) ST segment has nearly returned to the baseline.

The inverted T wave of ischemic heart disease (coronary insufficiency or myocardial infarction) has certain characteristic features. The T wave is symmetrical, the apex is midway between its two limbs and peaked like an arrowhead. The right and left sides of the inverted T wave of myocardial ischemia, are mirror images of each other **(Fig. 8.4)**.

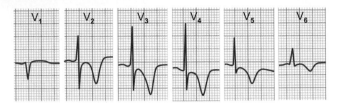

Fig. 8.4: Acute non-Q anterior wall myocardial infarction:
Convex ST segment; Symmetrical inverted T wave

A subtle evidence of myocardial ischemia is that the T wave amplitude in lead L_I is less than in L_{III} and that in lead V_6 is less than in V_1 **(Fig. 8.5)**.

Conditions associated with abnormal QRS morphology may also cause T wave inversion in the leads where the QRS complexes are upright. Three classical examples are ventricular hypertrophy, bundle branch block and WPW syndrome. The T wave inversion in these conditions is secondary to abnormal ventricular depolarization or intraventricular conduction and is called secondary T wave inversion.

The characteristic feature of secondary T wave inversion is that it is asymmetrical, with the distal limb steeper than the proximal limb and the apex is blunt **(Fig. 8.6)**.

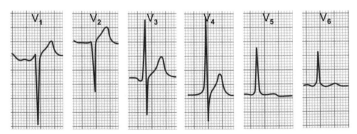

Fig. 8.5: Coronary insufficiency: T wave in V_1 taller than in V_6

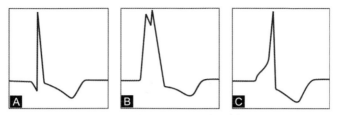

Fig. 8.6: Causes of secondary T wave inversion: (A) Ventricular hypertrophy; (B) Bundle branch block; (C) WPW syndrome

In left ventricular hypertrophy, the inverted T wave has a long and gradual downslope with a rapid return to the baseline, thus making it asymmetrical.

T wave inversion secondary to ventricular hypertrophy occurs in leads showing tall R waves. This along with S-T segment depression constitutes the pattern of systolic overload or ventricular strain **(Fig. 8.7A)**.

Mega-sized 'giant' inverted T waves are observed in hypertrophic cardiomyopathy where the hypertrophy is confined to the left ventricle apex. Similar deep inverted T waves are also seen after intracranial hemorrhage **(Fig. 8.7B)**.

In bundle branch block, the T wave is generally opposite to the direction of the QRS deflection and constitutes secondary T wave inversion. If the T wave is upright in leads showing

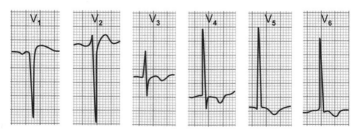

Fig. 8.7A: Left ventricular hypertrophy with strain: Depressed ST segment; Inverted T waves

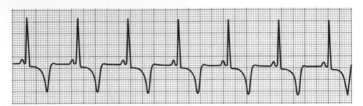

Fig. 8.7B: Hypertrophic apical cardiomyopathy: Giant inverted T waves

a positive QRS deflection, associated myocardial ischemia should be considered.

In WPW syndrome, the T wave is inverted in leads showing a wide and upright deflection. It reflects abnormal repolarization secondary to preexcitation of the ventricle.

T wave inversion in nearly all ECG leads is generally due to nonspecific causes, a metabolic abnormality or a diffuse process affecting the myocardium or pericardium. Regional inversion of the T wave in specific leads can be caused by specific etiological factors such as:

- *In leads L_I, aVL, V_5, V_6*
    - ⟹ Lateral wall ischemia/infarction
    - ⟹ Left ventricular hypertrophy
    - ⟹ Left bundle branch block
    - ⟹ Digitalis effect or toxicity.
- *In leads V_1, V_2, V_3*
    - ⟹ Anteroseptal ischemia/infarction
    - ⟹ Right ventricular hypertrophy
    - ⟹ Right bundle branch block
    - ⟹ WPW syndrome, type A
    - ⟹ Persistent juvenile pattern
    - ⟹ Acute pulmonary embolism
    - ⟹ Arrhythmogenic RV dysplasia.
- *In leads L_{II}, L_{III}, aVF*
    - ⟹ Inferior wall ischemia/infarction
    - ⟹ Mitral valve prolapse syndrome.

TALL T WAVE

The T wave exceeding a voltage of 5 mm in the standard leads and 10 mm in precordial leads is considered tall.

Causes of tall T waves are:

- Hyperkalemia **(Figs 8.8A and B)**
- Myocardial ischemia/injury
  - ➡ Hyperacute infarction
  - ➡ Prinzmetal's angina.

A high serum potassium value is classically associated with tall T waves. The T wave of hyperkalemia is very tall, peaked, symmetrical and has a narrow base, the so called 'tented' T wave **(Fig. 8.8A)**.

Other ECG features of hyperkalemia **(Fig. 8.8B)** depend upon serum potassium values and can be categorized as:

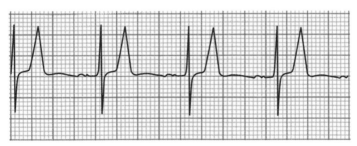

Fig. 8.8A: Effect of hyperkalemia on the T wave

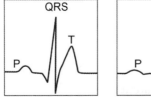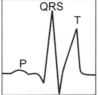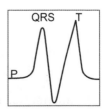

Fig. 8.8B: Effects of progressively increasing hyperkalemia

- Serum $K^+ > 6.8$ mEq/L
  - ➠ Tall tented T waves
  - ➠ Short QT interval
- Serum $K^+ > 8.4$ mEq/L
  - ➠ Low/absent P waves
- Serum K > 9.1 mEq/L
  - ➠ Wide, bizarre QRS
  - ➠ AV block and arrhythmias.

The common causes of hyperkalemia include renal failure, adrenal insufficiency, metabolic acidosis and excessive potassium intake. The clinical importance of hyperkalemia lies in the fact that it can cause life-threatening arrhythmias.

Since, hyperkalemia severe enough to cause gross ECG changes is most often due to renal failure, the clinical picture is usually that of uremia with hypertension, fluid overload, anemia and low urinary output.

Treatment of hyperkalemia includes elimination of dietary potassium, infusion of glucose with insulin, bicarbonate administration to combat acidosis, cation-exchange resins to bind potassium and hemodialysis in extreme situations.

In the hyperacute phase of myocardial infarction, there is ST segment elevation (convex upwards) along with tall T waves, the proximal limb of the T wave blending with the elevated ST segment **(Fig. 8.9)**.

This phase is followed by serial evolution of ECG changes with appearance of Q waves, settling down of the ST segment and inversion of the T waves. Because of myocardial necrosis secondary to coronary occlusion, the serum levels of cardiac enzymes (CPK, SGOT) are raised.

In a variety of angina called variant angina or Prinzmetal's angina, the basis of myocardial ischemia is not coronary thrombosis but coronary spasm. In such an ischemic episode of vasospastic angina, the ECG changes are similar to those

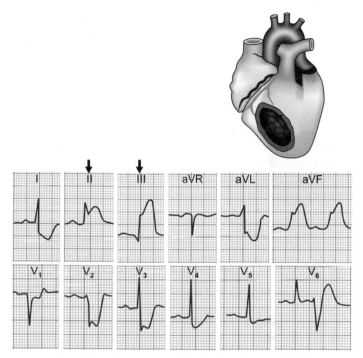

Fig. 8.9: Acute inferior myocardial infarction, hyperacute phase:
S-T elevation in II, III, aVF; Reciprocal depression in I, aVL

of hyperacute phase of infarction with S-T segment elevation and tall T waves **(Fig. 8.9)**.

The difference is that the ECG changes do not evolve serially but settle down rapidly. Q waves never appear and serum levels of cardiac enzymes are not raised as there is no myocardial necrosis.

Since the basis of Prinzmetal's angina is vasospasm, the coronary artery undergoing spasm can be predicted from the leads showing ECG changes, as depicted in **Table 8.1**.

TABLE 8.1: Relationship between location of ECG changes and coronary artery spasm

Coronary artery showing spasm of	Location of ECG changes
Left anterior descending artery	V_1, V_2, V_3, V_4
Left circumflex artery	L_I, aVL, V_5, V_6
Right coronary artery	L_{II}, L_{III}, aVF

The T wave may become excessively tall in the presence of coronary insufficiency. This T wave differs from the tall T wave of hyperkalemia, by the fact that it is broad based and the Q-T interval is prolonged. On the other hand in hyperkalemia, the T wave is narrow based or "tented" and the Q-T interval is shortened.

Abnormalities of the U Wave

NORMAL U WAVE

The U wave is produced by slow and late repolarization of the intraventricular Purkinje system and follows the T wave which represents repolarization of the main ventricular mass.

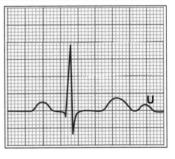

The normal U wave fulfills the following criteria:

- It is an upright deflection
- It is much smaller than the T wave.

It is often difficult to notice the U wave but when seen, it is best appreciated in the precordial leads V_2 to V_4. The U wave is easily visible when the QT interval is short, being clearly separated from the T wave it follows. It is also easily visible when the heart rate is slow, being clearly separated from the P wave that follows it.

PROMINENT U WAVE

A U wave that is exaggerated and approximates the size of the T wave, is considered to be a prominent U wave **(Fig. 9.1)**. The causes of prominent U waves are:

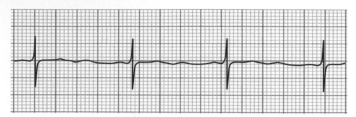

Fig. 9.1: Prominent U wave due to hypokalemia

- Hypokalemia and hypocalcemia
- Psychotropic tricyclic antidepressants
- Congenital long QT syndrome
- Early repolarization variant.

In hypokalemia, a prominent U wave that follows a low T wave produces a 'camel-hump' effect. Alternatively, a flat T wave followed by a prominent U wave may falsely suggest prolongation of the QT interval while actually it is the QU interval that is being measured.

Certain cardiovascular therapeutic agents and psycho-tropic drugs can cause prominence of the U waves. Knowledge of this fact can avoid the overdiagnosis of hypokalemia and QT interval prolongation.

INVERTED U WAVE

A U wave that is reversed in polarity is called an inverted U wave **(Fig. 9.2)**. The causes of inverted U wave are:
- Ischemic heart disease
- Left ventricular diastolic overload.

Inversion of U waves can be taken as a sign of myocar-dial ischemia or ventricular strain. When inversion is due to myocardial ischemia, this is usually associated with changes in the ST segment and T wave. Occasionally, U wave inversion may occur alone in the absence of ST-T changes.

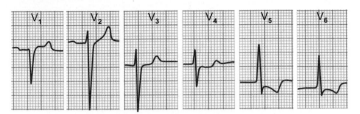

Fig. 9.2: Inverted U wave due to myocardial ischemia

Left ventricular overload may be systolic or diastolic. Inversion of the U wave occurs in diastolic (volume) overload. This is associated with tall QRS complexes in left ventricular leads V_5, V_6, L_I and aVL. The strain pattern of ST segment depression and T wave inversion is only observed in systolic (pressure) overload.

Abnormalities of PR Segment

All ECG deflections occur above or below a reference baseline known as the isoelectric line. The main segment of the isoelectric line intervenes between the T (or U) wave of one cardiac cycle and the P wave of the next cycle.

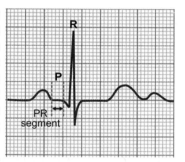

The portion of the isoelectric line between the termination of the P wave and the onset of the QRS complex is called the PR segment. It denotes the conduction delay in the atrioventricular node. Normally, the PR segment is at the same level as the main segment of the isoelectric line.

Potential abnormality of the PR segment is depression of the PR segment in relation to the baseline. Abnormalities of the length of the PR segment reflect variations in the duration of the PR interval.

PR SEGMENT DEPRESSION

The P wave is produced by atrial depolarization. The Ta wave is produced by atrial repolarization. Normally, the Ta wave is not seen as it coincides with and lies buried in the much

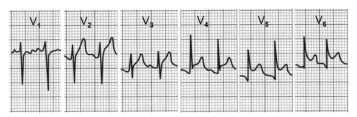

Fig. 10.1: Depressed PR segment due to acute pericarditis

larger QRS complex. Prominence of the Ta wave produces depression of the PR segment **(Fig. 10.1)**.

The causes of PR segment depression are:

- *Secondary causes*
  - Sinus tachycardia
  - Atrial enlargement
- *Primary causes*
  - Acute pericarditis
  - Atrial infarction
  - Chest wall trauma.

PR segment depression secondary to marked sinus tachycardia has no separate clinical relevance. A depressed PR segment alone has low sensitivity, as a diagnostic criteria for atrial enlargement.

Acute pericarditis is a frequent cause of PR segment depression and in fact, a diagnostic feature of this condition. In myocardial infarction, the PR segment is depressed only if atrial infarction occurs. This fact is used to differentiate acute pericarditis from acute myocardial infarction since both conditions present with chest pain and ECG changes.

Depression of the PR segment may follow trauma to the chest wall, either accidental or surgical. The PR segment depression observed after penetrating chest wounds or cardiac surgery, is due to accompanying pericarditis or atrial injury.

Abnormalities of ST Segment

All ECG deflections occur above or below a reference baseline known as the isoelectric line. The main segment of the isoelectric line intervenes between the T (or U) wave of one cardiac cycle and the P wave of the next cycle.

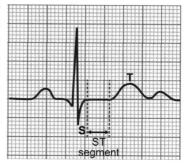

The portion of the isoelectric line between the termination of the S wave (J point) and the onset of the T wave is called the ST segment. It represents the slow plateau phase of ventricular repolarization. Normally, the ST segment is at the same level as the main segment of the isoelectric line.

Potential abnormalities of the ST segment are depression or elevation of the ST segment in relation to the baseline. Abnormalities of the length of the ST segment reflect variation in the duration of the QT interval.

ST SEGMENT DEPRESSION

Depression of the ST segment greater than 1.0 mm in relation to the baseline constitutes significant ST segment depression. Since depression of the ST segment is often associated with inversion of the T wave, together they are referred to as ST-T changes.

The causes of ST segment depression are:

Nonspecific causes

- *Physiological states*
  - ⇒ Anxiety
  - ⇒ Tachycardia
  - ⇒ Hyperventilation
- *Extracardiac disorders*
  - ⇒ Systemic, e.g. hemorrhage, shock
  - ⇒ Cranial, e.g. cerebrovascular accident
  - ⇒ Abdominal, e.g. pancreatitis, cholecystitis
  - ⇒ Respiratory, e.g. pulmonary embolism.

Specific causes

- *Primary abnormality*
  - ⇒ Pharmacological, e.g. digitalis, quinidine
  - ⇒ Metabolic, e.g. hypokalemia, hypothermia
  - ⇒ Myocardial, e.g. cardiomyopathy, myocarditis
  - ⇒ Ischemic, e.g. coronary insufficiency, infarction.
- *Secondary abnormality*
  - ⇒ Ventricular hypertrophy
  - ⇒ Bundle branch block
  - ⇒ WPW syndrome.

ST segment depression lacks specificity as a diagnostic indicator. Since depression of the ST segment can be caused by certain physiological states and noncardiac diseases, it only highlights the importance of viewing any ECG finding in the light of clinical data.

One should be careful before diagnosing myocardial ischemia only by ECG criteria. ST segment depression should be interpreted with caution in upper abdominal and respiratory diseases where the clinical picture may be confused with that of heart disease.

Digitalis administration produces various ECG abnormalities of which ST segment depression is an important manifestation. The depressed ST segment either assumes a shape that is a mirror-image of the correction tick ($\sqrt{}$) **(Fig. 11.1)**.

When these changes are confined to leads V_5, V_6, they indicate digitalis administration. Changes occurring in most leads are suggestive of digitalis intoxication.

Hypokalemia causes ST segment depression **(Fig. 11.2)** but the more prominent abnormalities are:

- Low or flat T waves
- Prominent U waves
- Prolonged PR interval
- Prolonged QU interval

Primary diseases of the myocardium, such as cardio-myopathy and acute myocarditis produce ST segment depression and T wave inversion. These changes are often associated with wide QRS complexes due to intraventricular conduction defect.

Clinically speaking, coronary artery disease is the most important cause of ST segment depression. In myocardial ischemia, the degree of ST segment depression (greater than 1 mm) generally correlates with severity of coronary insufficiency **(Fig. 11.3)**.

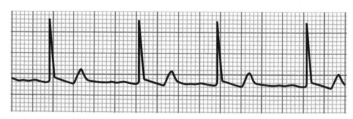

Fig. 11.1: Effect of digitalis on the ST segment

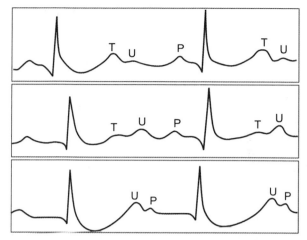

Fig. 11.2: Effects of progressively increasing hypokalemia

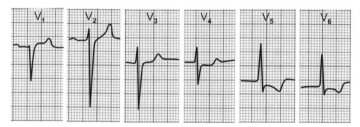

Fig. 11.3: Lateral wall ischemic changes after angina pectoris: Depression of ST segment; inversion of T wave

Besides being depressed, the morphology of the ST segment associated with increasing severity of myocardial ischemia, can be classified as given in **Figure 11.4**.

In acute coronary insufficiency, the ST segment acquires a coved or convex appearance. This change may be observed in several leads in contrast to localized changes seen in regional myocardial ischemia. Acute non-Q myocardial infarction may also produce an identical picture **(Fig. 11.5)** but with the following differences:

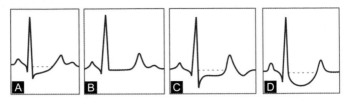

Fig. 11.4: Types of ST segment depression with increasing severity of myocardial ischemia: (A) Only J point depression (upsloping ST segment); (B) Horizontality of ST segment (sharp ST-T junction); (C) Plane ST depression (horizontal ST depression); (D) Sagging depression (hammock-like ST segment)

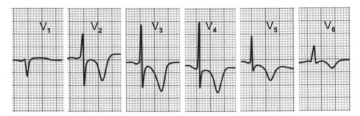

Fig. 11.5: Acute non-Q anterior wall myocardial infarction:
Convex ST segment; inverted T wave

- There is history of prolonged chest pain
- Cardiac enzymes (e.g. CPK) are raised
- ST-T changes persist in serial ECGs.

In acute Q-wave myocardial infarction, the ECG leads oriented towards the infarct show ST segment elevation while the leads oriented towards the uninjured surface of the heart may reveal ST segment depression. Such depression of the ST segment is termed as reciprocal depression.

For instance, inferior wall myocardial infarction leads to ST segment elevation in leads L_{II} L_{III} and aVF, while leads L_I and aVL show ST segment depression **(Fig. 11.6)**.

Depression of the ST segment constitutes the most useful criterion for the positivity of the exercise ECG test (stress test) using a treadmill or bicycle egometer. The degree of positivity

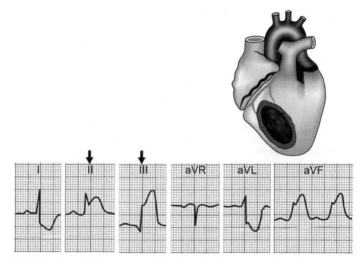

Fig. 11.6:   Acute inferior myocardial infarction, hyperacute phase: ST elevation in II, III, aVF; reciprocal depression in I, aVL

of the stress test (mild, moderate or severe) can be gauged from these parameters of ST segment depression:

Degree of ST Depression

Greater the magnitude of ST depression, higher is the grade of positivity of the stress test. A depression of 3 mm or more indicates severe coronary artery disease.

Nature of ST Depression

The types of ST depression with increasing diagnostic significance are:

➠ Rapid upstroke of ST segment
➠ Slow upstroke of ST segment
➠ Horizontal ST segment depression
➠ Downslope ST segment depression.

Timing of ST Depression

Earlier the appearance of ST depression in the exercise period, greater is the grade of positivity of the stress test. Depression that appears in the first stage of exercise indicates greater positivity than that which appears in the third stage.

Duration of ST Depression

Greater the total duration of ST depression (exercise plus recovery period), more is the grade of positivity of the stress test. Depression that persists for up to 8 minutes of the recovery period indicates severe coronary disease.

Conditions associated with abnormal QRS morphology may also cause ST segment depression in the leads where the QRS complex is upright. Three classical examples are ventricular hypertrophy, bundle branch block and WPW syndrome. The ST segment depression in these conditions is secondary to an abnormality of ventricular depolarization or intraventricular conduction and is called secondary ST segment depression.

Secondary ST segment depression can be differentiated from primary depression of myocardial ischemia by the shape of the T wave. The T wave of ischemia is symmetrical and peaked while that of secondary ST depression is asymmetrical and blunt **(Fig. 11.7)**.

ST SEGMENT ELEVATION

Elevation of the ST segment exceeding 1 mm in relation to the baseline constitutes significant ST segment elevation. The causes of ST segment elevation are:
- Coronary artery disease
    - ⇛ Myocardial infarction
    - ⇛ Prinzmetal's angina
    - ⇛ Dressler's syndrome

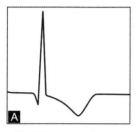 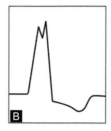 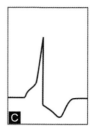

Fig. 11.7: Causes of secondary ST depression: (A) Ventricular hypertrophy;
(B) Bundle branch block; (C) WPW syndrome

- Acute pericarditis
- Ventricular aneurysm
- Early repolarization.

Acute myocardial infarction is the most common and clinically the most significant cause of ST segment elevation (ST elevation myocardial infarction—STEMI). In the hyperacute phase of infarction, the elevated ST segment slopes upwards to blend smoothly with the proximal limb of the T wave. In this stage, the T wave is upright and the Q wave is not observed. In the evolved phase, the elevated ST segment becomes convex upwards, the T wave gets symmetrically inverted, the Q wave appears and there is loss of R wave height **(Fig. 11.8)**.

The age of a myocardial infarct can be related to the stage of ECG changes as follows:

- Acute MI   0 hour to 6 hours
- Recent MI   7 hours to 7 days
- Evolved MI   8 days to 28 days
- Healed MI   More than 29 days

The leads which show ST segment elevation in myocardial infarction depend upon the location of the infarct and can be expressed as given in **Table 11.1**.

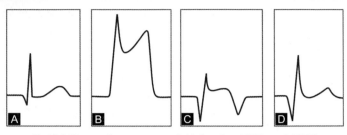

Fig. 11.8: Phases of acute myocardial infarction: (A) Normal QRS-T; (B) Hyperacute phase; (C) Fully evolved phase; (D) Stabilized phase

TABLE 11.1: Location of infarction determined from ECG leads

ST elevation in	Location of infarction
V_1 to V_4	Anteroseptal
V_1, V_2	Septal
V_3, V_4	Anterior
L_I, aVL	High lateral
V_5-V_6 L_I aVL	Lateral
V_3-V_6 L_I aVL	Anterolateral
V_1-V_6 L_I aVL	Extensive anterior
L_{II} L_{III} avF	Inferior
V_3R V_4R	Right ventricular

Besides ST segment elevation, other electrocardiographic features of myocardial infarction are:

- Symmetrical T wave inversion
- Appearance of Q wave
- Loss of R wave height
- Regional location of changes
- Reciprocal ST depression in other leads
- Arrhythmias and conduction defects
- Serial evolution of ECG changes.

The ECG findings of a myocardial infarct depend upon several factors, such as:

- Age of the infarct; hyperacute or recent damage
- Type of the infarct; transmural or subendocardial
- Site of the infarct; anterior wall or inferior wall
- Underlying abnormality; LBBB, LVH or WPW.

Reasons for disparity between ECG changes and clinical findings include:

- Left circumflex disease
- Attenuation phenomenon
- Hibernating myocardium
- Mechanical complication.

In Prinzmetal's angina, the ECG changes are very similar to those of the hyperacute phase of myocardial infarction with the following differences:

- ECG changes resolve rapidly and do not evolve serially
- Serum levels of cardiac enzymes (e.g. CPK) are normal.

The basis of Prinzmetal's angina is coronary spasm and not coronary thrombosis as in the case of myocardial infarction. Coronary spasm may be provoked by injection of intracoronary ergonovine. The coronary artery undergoing spasm can be predicted from the leads showing ST elevation as shown in **Table 11.2**.

Besides acute myocardial infarction, another frequent cause of ST segment elevation is acute pericarditis. Since both these conditions are associated with chest pain, given the

TABLE 11.2: Relationship between location of ST elevation and coronary artery spasm

ST elevation in	Coronary artery spasm of
V_1, V_2, V_3, V_4	Left anterior descending artery
V_5, V_6, L_1, avL	Left circumflex artery
L_{II}, L_{III}, avF	Right coronary artery

more serious nature of myocardial infarction, it is extremely important to differentiate them.

Electrocardiographic features of acute pericarditis **(Fig. 11.9)**, as different from those of acute myocardial infarction are:

- ST segment elevation is flat or concave upwards
- ST elevation is observed in nearly all leads
- T wave is upright and elevated off the baseline
- Q wave does not appear at any stage
- R wave height is maintained
- PR segment is depressed
- There is no reciprocal ST segment depression
- Sinus tachycardia is almost invariably present
- Arrhythmias and conduction defects are unusual
- ECG changes do not evolve but resolve rapidly.

During the resolving phase of acute myocardial infarction, occasionally, there may be re-elevation of the ST segment for which three explanations may be offered.

- Firstly, it may be due to reinfarction with re-elevation of cardiac enzymes requiring intensive treatment
- Secondly, it may represent coronary vasospasm, the significance of which is similar to that of Prinzmetal's angina
- Finally, ST segment re-elevation may be due to the post-infarction syndrome or Dressler syndrome.

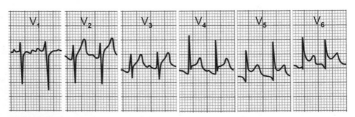

Fig. 11.9: Acute pericarditis: Saddle-shaped ST segment elevation

The specific features of Dressler syndrome are:

- Elevation of ST segment without reciprocal depression
- Precordial pain increasing on inspiration
- Fever and tachycardia are often present
- Raised ESR but normal cardiac enzymes
- Appearance of pleuropericardial rub
- Responsiveness to steroid therapy.

A picture similar to that in Dressler's syndrome may be observed in the postcardiotomy syndrome that follows cardiac surgery, chest wall trauma or pacemaker implant.

Any survivor of myocardial infarction in whom the typical pattern of the evolved phase of infarction persists for three months or longer after acute attack, should be suspected to have developed a ventricular aneurysm.

However, this ECG sign has a low sensitivity for the diagnosis of an aneurysm. The presence of a ventricular aneurysm has to be confirmed by echocardiography.

There exists a benign but often alarming electrocardiographic entity that presents with concave upward S-T segment elevation and an entirely normal clinical profile. It is known as the "early repolarization" syndrome. Since it is observed in young healthy individuals, this entity is also known as the "athletic heart".

It represents early repolarization of a portion of the myocardium, before the entire myocardium has been depolarized.

There is an early uptake of the ST segment before the descending limb of the R wave has reached the baseline. This causes an initial slur on the ST segment known as the J wave. The J wave or Osborne wave is also observed in hypothermia.

The T waves are tall and upright in the lateral leads and the U waves are prominent in the mid-precordial leads **(Fig. 11.10)**.

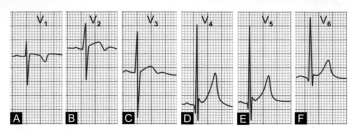

Fig. 11.10: ECG features of early repolarization syndrome: (A) Tall R waves in leads V4 to V6; (B) Deep and narrow initial q waves; (C) Concave-upward ST segment elevation; (D) Initial slur on ST segment; the J wave; (E) Tall and upright symmetrical T waves; (F) Prominent mid-precordial U waves

Other ECG features of the athletic heart are:
- Sinus bradycardia with sinus arrhythmia
- Voltage criteria of left ventricular hypertrophy
- Persistent juvenile pattern (T wave inversion V_1 to V_3).

The clinical features of early repolarization syndrome are:
- Subject is a young black male
- He is healthy and of athletic built
- He is active and free from symptoms
- The clinical evaluation is entirely normal
- ST segment returns to baseline after exercise.

Abnormalities of PR Interval

NORMAL PR INTERVAL

The PR interval is measured on the horizontal axis from the onset of the P wave to the beginning of the QRS complex, irrespective of whether it begins with a Q wave or R wave. The width of the P wave is included in the length of PR interval.

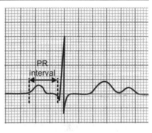

Since the P wave represents atrial depolarization and the QRS complex represents ventricular depolarization, the PR interval is a measure of the atrioventricular (AV) conduction time. The AV conduction time includes the time taken for atrial depolarization, the conduction delay in the AV node and the time taken for an impulse to traverse the intraventricular conduction system before ventricular depolarization begins.

Since the conduction delay in the AV node is the major fraction of the PR interval, the length of PR interval is a measure of the duration of AV nodal delay.

The normal PR interval in adults ranges from 0.12 to 0.20 second depending upon the heart rate. It is longer at slow heart rates and shorter at fast heart rates. The PR interval is slightly shorter in children, the upper limit being 0.18 second. It is slightly longer in the elderly, the upper limit being 0.22 second.

Potential abnormalities of the PR interval are:

- Prolonged PR interval
- Shortened PR interval
- Variable PR interval.

PROLONGED PR INTERVAL

A PR interval that exceeds 0.20 second in adults and 0.18 second in children is taken as prolonged. Since the PR interval reflects atrioventricular conduction time, a prolonged PR interval indicates increased AV nodal conduction delay or first degree atrioventricular (AV) block **(Fig. 12.1)**.

The causes of prolonged PR interval are:

- Vagal dominance in athletes
- Acute rheumatic fever or diphtheria
- Coronary artery disease with fascicular block
- Drugs acting on the AV node, e.g. digitalis, beta-blockers, calcium-channel blockers.

PR interval prolongation is normally observed in vago-tonic individuals, such as athletes. It is also a normal effect of vagal stimulation, e.g. carotid sinus massage and sympathetic blockade, e.g. beta-blocker administration.

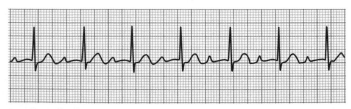

Fig. 12.1: Prolonged PR interval: First-degree AV block

A prolonged PR interval is one of the diagnostic criteria of acute rheumatic fever and indicates carditis. Similarly, a prolonged PR interval in diphtheria indicates myocarditis.

PR interval prolongation is usual with cardiovascular drugs that act on the AV node and delay AV conduction. Examples are digitalis, verapamil, diltiazem, propranolol and metoprolol.

Prolongation of the PR interval in the presence of bundle branch block indicates that atrioventricular conduction down the unblocked bundle branch is also delayed. Since such patients are likely to develop complete AV block, they may require prophylactic cardiac pacing.

SHORTENED PR INTERVAL

A PR interval that is less than 0.12 second is considered short. Since PR interval reflects atrioventricular conduction time, a short PR interval indicates decreased AV nodal delay. The causes of shortened PR interval are:

- AV nodal or junctional rhythm
- WPW syndrome with pre-excitation
- Drugs that hasten AV conduction.

If a cardiac rhythm originates from the AV nodal area (junctional rhythm), the ventricles are activated in the normal sequence but the atria are activated retrogradely, that is, from below upwards. Since the atria are activated nearly simultaneously with the ventricles, the P waves just precede, just follow or are merged in the QRS complexes. When the P waves just precede the QRS complexes, they are associated with a short PR interval (**Fig. 12.2**).

A junctional rhythm at its inherent discharge rate of 40–60 beats per minute constitutes a junctional escape rhythm while a junctional rhythm at an enhanced rate of 60–100 beats per minute constitutes a junctional tachycardia.

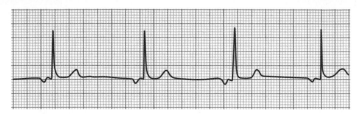

Fig. 12.2: Shortened PR interval: Junctional rhythm

The Wolff-Parkinson-White (WPW) syndrome is an entity in which an accessory pathway or bypass tract called the bundle of Kent directly connects the atrial to the ventricular myocardium without passing through the AV node. Fast conduction of impulses down this tract results in premature ventricular activation called pre-excitation, since the AV node is bypassed. This results in a short PR interval **(Fig. 12.3)**.

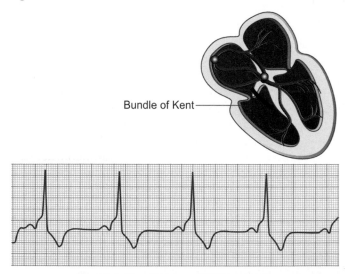

Bundle of Kent

Fig. 12.3: Short PR interval: WPW syndrome

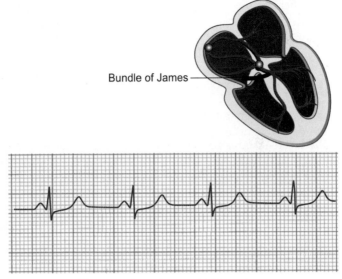

Fig. 12.4: Short PR interval: LGL syndrome

The QRS complex is wide because it is a fusion beat which is the blend of ventricular pre-excitation (by bundle of Kent) and normal ventricular activation (by bundle of His). Pre-excitation causes a slur on the ascending limb or R wave known as the delta wave. ST segment depression and T wave inversion are secondary ST-T changes.

In the Lown-Ganong-Levine (LGL) syndrome, an accessory atriofascicular tract (James bypass) directly connects the atria to the bundle of His. This causes pre-excitation of the ventricles and a short PR interval without AV nodal delay. The QRS complex is narrow because the ventricles are activated as usual by the bundle of His **(Fig. 12.4)**.

The PR interval is prolonged in vagotonic individuals and with vagal stimulation. Conversely, the PR interval is shortened with vagolytic drugs, e.g. atropine and other drugs that have anticholinergic effects.

VARIABLE PR INTERVAL

During any rhythm, a changing PR interval on a beat-to-beat basis is designated as variable PR interval. Normally, atrial activation (P wave) is followed by ventricular activation (QRS complex) with an identical intervening PR interval in all beats, thus establishing fixed relationship between them.

If atrial and ventricular activation occur independent of each other and not sequentially, or if the extent of AV nodal conduction delay varies from beat-to-beat, the PR interval is variable.

The causes of variable PR interval are:
- Type I, second-degree AV block
- Junctional pacemaker rhythm
- Complete, third-degree AV block
- Wandering pacemaker rhythm
- Multifocal atrial tachycardia.

Abnormalities of QT Interval

NORMAL QT INTERVAL

The QT interval is measured on the horizontal axis from the onset of the Q wave to the termination of the T wave (not the U wave). The duration of the QRS complex, the length of the ST segment and the width of the T wave are included in the measurement of the QT interval.

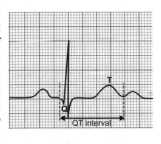

Since the QRS duration represents ventricular depolarization time and the T wave width represents ventricular repolarization time the QT interval is a measure of the total duration of ventricular electrical systole.

The normal QT interval is in the range of 0.35–0.43 second or 0.39 ± 0.04 second. The upper limit of normal QT interval depends upon several variables including age, gender, autonomic tone and drug therapy.

The QT interval tends to be shorter in young individuals (<0.44 second) and slightly longer in the elderly (<0.45 sec). It is slightly shorter in males, the upper limit being 0.43 sec. The QT interval shortens at fast heart rates and lengthens at slow heart rates.

Therefore, for proper interpretation, the QT interval must be corrected for the heart rate. The corrected QT interval is known as the QTc interval. The QTc interval is determined using the Bazett's formula:

$$QTc = \frac{QT}{\sqrt{RR}}$$

QT is the measured QT interval

$\sqrt{RR}$ is square-root of RR interval

When the RR interval is 25 mm or 1 second (25 × 0.04 second = 1 second), the value of $\sqrt{RR}$ is 1 and the QTc is equal to the QT interval. This occurs at a heart rate of 60 beats/min.

As a general rule, QT interval than exceeds half of the duration of RR interval is taken as prolonged.

Potential abnormalities of the QT interval are:
- Shortened QT interval
- Prolonged QT interval.

SHORTENED QT INTERVAL

A corrected QT interval (QTc interval) less than 0.35 second is considered short **(Fig. 13.1)**. The causes of a shortened QTc interval are:
- Hyperkalemia
- Hypercalcemia
- Digitalis effect

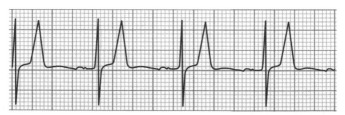

Fig. 13.1: Shortened QT interval due to hyperkalemia

- Acidosis
- Hyperthermia.

Hyperkalemia shortens the QT interval and is associated with tall T waves, wide QRS complexes and diminished P waves. Hypercalcemia also shortens the QT interval but there are no changes in the morphology of the QRS deflection or of the P and T waves.

A short QT interval with ST segment depression and T wave inversion suggests digitalis effect. Antiarrhythmic drugs also produce ST-T changes but the QT interval is prolonged.

PROLONGED QT INTERVAL

A corrected QT interval (QTc interval) greater than 0.43 second is considered prolonged **(Fig. 13.2)**. The causes of a prolonged QTc interval can be classified as:

- Congenital QT syndromes
  - ⮕ Romano-Ward syndrome (autosomal dominant, without deafness)
  - ⮕ Jerwell-Lange-Nielson syndrome (autosomal recessive, with deafness).
- Acquired QT syndromes
  - ⮕ Electrolyte deficiency, e.g. potassium, calcium
  - ⮕ Antiarrhythmic drugs, e.g. quinidine, amiodarone
  - ⮕ Coronary disease, e.g. acute myocardial infarction
  - ⮕ Acute myocarditis, e.g. viral myocarditis, rheumatic fever

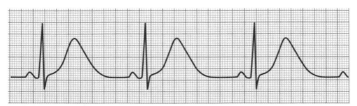

Fig. 13.2: Prolonged QT interval due to amiodarone

➠ Intracranial event, e.g. head injury, hemorrhage
➠ Bradyarrhythmias, e.g. AV block, sinus bradycardia
➠ Psychotropic drugs, e.g. tricyclic antidepressants
➠ Miscellaneous drugs, e.g. terfenadine, cisapride.

Hypocalcemia produces true prolongation of the QT interval without any alteration of the ST segment or T wave.

In hypokalemia, the T wave is flattened and the prominent U wave may be mistaken for the T wave. This may falsely suggest prolongation of the QT interval, whereas it is actually the QU interval. Hypokalemia, therefore, causes pseudo-prolongation of the QT interval **(Fig. 13.3)**.

Antiarrhythmic drugs, such as quinidine, procainamide and amiodarone can prolong the QT interval. They also cause widening of the QRS complex which if exceeds 25% of baseline, is an indication for withdrawing the culprit drug.

Since QT interval prolongation predisposes to arrhythmias, this is one way to explain the arrhythmia enhancing property or proarrhythmic effect of antiarrhythmic drugs.

Certain noncardiovascular drugs, such as the anti-histamine terfenadine and the prokinetic cisapride prolong the QT interval. They do so especially in combination with ketoconazole (antifungal), erythromycin (macrolide antibiotic) or a statin (cholesterol lowering drug), which also utilize the same cytochrome enzyme CYP3A4 for hepatic metabolism. Therefore, it is mandatory to measure

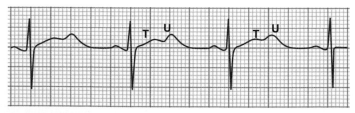

Fig. 13.3: Pseudo-prolonged QT interval in hypokalemia

the QT interval, in clinical trials undertaken for new drug development.

The clinical importance of QT interval prolongation lies in the fact that it predisposes to a typical type of polymorphic ventricular arrhythmia known as "Torsade de pointes" a ballet term which literally means "torsion around a point".

This term explains the morphology ot the ventricular tachycardia which consists of polymorphic QRS complexes that keep changing in amplitude and direction. The polymorphic QRS complexes give the appearance of torsion or twisting of points around the isoelectric line.

Besides QT prolongation and Torsade de pointes, other features of long QT syndrome (LQTS) are T wave alternans and notched T waves.

Premature Beats in Regular Rhythm

PREMATURE BEATS

Premature beats are impulses that arise due to the premature firing of an irritable automaticity focus other than the normal pacemaker, the SA node. They are also known as premature contractions, premature complexes or simply extrasystole.

According to focus of origin, premature beats are classified as:
- Atrial premature beats
- Junctional premature beats
- Ventricular premature beats.

Atrial and junctional premature complexes are together referred to as supraventricular premature beats.

ATRIAL PREMATURE COMPLEX

An atrial premature complex (APC) **(Fig. 14.1)** is recognized by the following features:
- Premature inscription of an upright P wave, earlier than the expected sinus P wave
- Abnormal morphology of the premature P wave due to ectopic focus of origin
- Normal morphology of the QRS complex that follows it, since ventricular conduction is normal
- Compensatory pause after the APC due to momentary suppression of SA node automaticity.

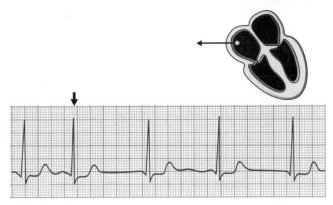

Fig. 14.1: Atrial premature beat: Ectopic P wave, narrow QRS,
incomplete compensatory pause

Occasionally, two variations of APCs may be observed:

- *Blocked APC:* A very premature APC may find the AV node still refractory to ventricular conduction and may consequently get blocked. Such an APC inscribes a P wave that deforms the T wave of the preceding beat, is not followed by a QRS complex but is followed by a compensatory pause
- *APC with aberrant ventricular conduction:* Most often, the QRS complex of the APC is normal in morphology. However, if the APC finds one of the bundle branches still refractory to ventricular conduction, it inscribes a wide QRS complex or bundle branch block pattern. This is known as aberrant ventricular conduction of the APC.

APCs alternating with sinus impulses constitute a bigeminal rhythm (extrasystolic atrial bigeminy) while a series of three or more successive APCs constitute an atrial tachycardia. Frequent APCs arising from different atrial foci constitute a multifocal atrial tachycardia.

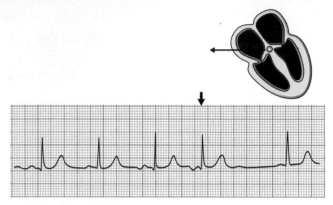

Fig. 14.2: Junctional premature beat: Inverted P wave, narrow QRS, incomplete compensatory pause

JUNCTIONAL PREMATURE COMPLEX

A junctional premature complex (JPC) **(Fig. 14.2)** is very similar to an APC but with these differences:

- The P wave of the JPC if seen, is inverted because of retrograde atrial activation
- The P wave just precedes, just follows or is merged in the QRS complex because of near simultaneous atrial and ventricular activation.

Since, both atrial and junctional premature complexes have a somewhat similar clinical relevance and are managed in the same way, their differentiation is often futile and they are together referred to as supraventricular premature complexes.

VENTRICULAR PREMATURE COMPLEX

A ventricular premature complex (VPC) **(Fig. 14.3)** is recognized by the following features:

- Premature inscription of a QRS complex earlier than the next expected sinus beat

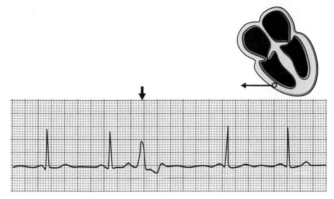

Fig. 14.3: Ventricular premature beat: Absent P wave, wide QRS, complete compensatory pause

- Wide and bizarre morphology of the QRS complex due to slow activation of the ventricles
- Bizarre QRS complex is not preceded by a P wave because of ventricular origin of the beat. A sinus P wave even if it occurs independently, is not visible as it is buried in the wide QRS complex
- Compensatory pause after the VPC. When a VPC is inscribed, a sinus beat that was to occur around that time is missed but the next sinus beat is inscribed as usual. This is expressed as a compensatory pause after the VPC. The compensatory pause after a VPC is complete, that is, it fully compensates for the prematurity of the VPC. This is in contrast to an APC where the compensatory pause is incomplete and the next sinus beat is only somewhat delayed.

On the basis of their occurrence, VPCs can be qualified as:

- VPCs of different morphology and varying coupling interval (between VPC and preceding sinus beat) are known as multifocal VPCs **(Fig. 14.4)**

- VPCs of similar morphology and constant coupling interval are known as unifocal VPCs **(Fig. 14.5)**
- VPC occurring late in the diastolic period of the preceding sinus beat (long coupling interval), just about when the next sinus beat is due, is called an end-diastolic VPC
- VPC that is so premature (very short coupling interval) that it is imposed upon the T wave of the preceding sinus impulse, exhibits the R-on-T phenomenon **(Fig. 14.6)**.

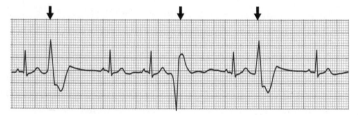

Fig. 14.4: Multifocal VPCs: Different morphology, variable coupling interval

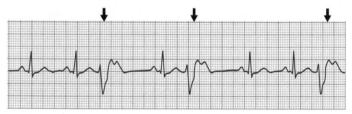

Fig. 14.5: Unifocal VPCs: Similar morphology, constant coupling interval

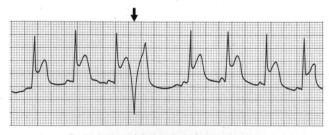

Fig. 14.6: VPC exhibiting R-on-T phenomenon:
Deformed T wave of preceding beat

- VPC during a slow rhythm, that does not allow any sinus beat to be missed and is not followed by a compensatory pause, is called an interpolated VPC **(Fig. 14.7)**. It appears to be sandwiched between two sinus beats
- VPCs alternating with sinus beats constitute a bigeminal rhythm (extrasystolic ventricular bigeminy) **(Fig. 14.8)**. VPCs after every two sinus beats represent trigeminy **(Fig. 14.9)** and after every third sinus beat constitute quadrigeminy
- A pair of successive VPCs form a couplet **(Fig. 14.10)** and three consecutive VPCs constitute a triplet **(Fig. 14.11)**.

A VPC is quite different in morphology from an APC, the former having a wide and bizarre QRS complex while the latter possessing a narrow QRS complex. Their differentiation assumes importance only if an APC conducts aberrantly to the ventricles and inscribes a wide QRS complex.

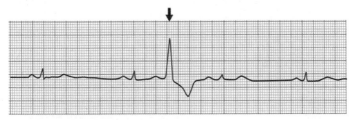

Fig. 14.7: Interpolated VPC: Ectopic beat sandwiched between two sinus beats

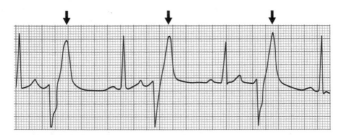

Fig. 14.8: Extrasystolic ventricular bigeminy: VPCs alternating with sinus beats

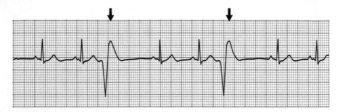

Fig. 14.9: Extrasystolic ventricular trigeminy: VPC after every two sinus beats

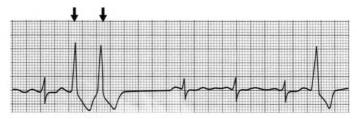

Fig. 14.10: Couplet of ventricular ectopic beats: Two VPCs in succession

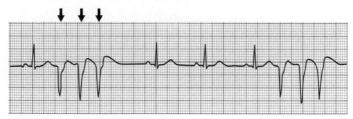

Fig. 14.11: Triplet of ventricular ectopic beats: Three VPCs in succession

An APC with aberrant ventricular conduction can be differentiated from a true VPC by the following features:
- Preceding P wave
- Triphasic QRS contour
- Incomplete compensatory pause.

Clinical Relevance of Premature Complexes

Supraventricular Premature Complexes

Atrial premature complexes (APCs) are common even in normal persons and occur due to these causes:

- Emotional stress or physical exercise
- Smoking or high intake of tea/coffee
- Drugs, e.g. salbutamol, theophylline
- Metabolic causes, e.g. hypoxia, acidosis.

Junctional premature complexes (JPCs) are less common than APCs and are less likely to occur in normal persons. In other words, their presence is more indicative of heart disease. Cardiac causes of APCs and JPCs are:

- Rheumatic carditis
- Digitalis toxicity
- Myocardial infarction
- Pericarditis
- Thyrotoxicosis
- Cardiac surgery.

Although APCs may be asymptomatic, the most common symptoms due to them are palpitations and sensation of "missed beats". JPCs cause similar symptoms but additionally produce neck-pulsation because of synchronous atrial and ventricular contraction or atrial contraction during AV valve closure.

Treatment of supraventricular premature complexes is generally not required especially if they are asymptomatic and not associated with organic heart disease. Management is indicated if premature beats are frequent enough to produce symptoms or if they trigger tachyarrhythmias, such as supraventricular tachycardia or atrial flutter.

The first step in management is avoidance of precipitating factors, such as stress, vigorous exercise, smoking, beverage consumption and adrenergic drugs. Addition of a mild sedative may be useful in some patients. The next step is treatment of any underlying cardiac condition, if present. This includes withdrawal of digitalis, treatment of rheumatic fever, control of thyrotoxicosis and management of ischemia.

If premature beats are frequent, low doses of beta-blockers or diltiazem are effective in controlling the ventricular rate. Propranolol may be the drug of choice in the management of premature beats caused by anxiety, adrenergic drugs and other catecholamine excess states. Amiodarone is quite effective in suppressing the ectopic atrial focus.

Ventricular Premature Complexes

Ventricular premature complexes (VPCs) can occur even in normal individuals although they are more often due to organic heart disease.

Causes of VPCs in normal persons are:
- Emotional stress or physical exercise
- Smoking or high intake of tea/coffee
- Drugs, e.g. sympathomimetics, theophylline
- Anxiety neurosis or thyrotoxicosis.

Cardiac conditions where VPCs are observed are:
- *Coronary artery disease*
  - ⇒ Ischemia
  - ⇒ Infarction
  - ⇒ Reperfusion.
- *Congestive heart failure*
  - ⇒ Hypertension
  - ⇒ Cardiomyopathy
  - ⇒ Myocarditis
  - ⇒ Ventricular aneurysm
- *Mitral valve prolapse syndrome*
- *Digitalis treatment/intoxication*
- *Cardiac surgery or catheterization.*

VPCs that meet the following criteria are considered to be "dangerous" or "malignant" VPCs.

- Occurring frequently (6 or more beats/minute)
- In showers with runs of ventricular tachycardia
- In couplets or VPCs in bigeminal rhythm
- With short coupling interval (R-on-T phenomenon)
- More than 0.14 second wide, bizarre or multifocal
- Associated with serious organic heart disease and left ventricular dysfunction.

Severity of ventricular ectopy can be classified on the basis of Lown's classification, as given in **Table 14.1**.

Multifocal VPCs arise from different irritable ventricular foci, each producing a distinctive VPC, every time it fires. Since even a single irritable focus can fire a salvo of rapid discharges to cause ventricular tachycardia, presence of multifocal VPCs means that several foci are discharging and trouble is imminent. The chances of developing life-threatening ventricular fibrillation are enhanced.

A VPC that occurs very prematurely (very short coupling interval) superimposes on the T wave of the preceding sinus beat and is said to exhibit the 'R-on-T' phenomenon. This represents the occurrence of ventricular stimulation during the vulnerable phase of Purkinje fiber repolarization or

TABLE 14.1: Lown's classification of ventricular ectopy

Category	Degree of ectopy
Class 0	No ectopy
Class 1	Less than 30/hour
Class 2	More than 30/hour
Class 3	Multiform VPCs
Class 4A	Couplets
Class 4B	Runs of 3 or more
Class 5	R-on-T phenomenon

period of heightened excitability and is likely to precipitate ventricular fibrillation.

The 'R-on-T' phenomenon is observed in:

- VPCs after acute myocardial infarction
- VPCs with underlying QT interval prolongation
- Electrical cardioversion during digitalis therapy
- Very premature stimuli during artificial pacing.

Ventricular premature complexes (VPCs) may be asymptomatic or associated with palpitations and sensation of "missed beats". Awareness of VPCs is due to the post-VPC compensatory pause and increased force of contraction of the beat following the VPC.

Neck pulsations may be felt due to atrial systole occurring with a closed tricuspid valve as the atria and ventricles are activated almost synchronously by the VPC.

Management of VPCs is governed by:

- Symptoms produced by premature beats
- Presence or absence of organic heart disease
- Nature and severity of ventricular ectopy.

Few isolated asymptomatic VPCs, in the absence of heart disease, are mostly left alone. If they are symptomatic, a search for etiological factors must be made and they should be corrected adequately.

Such measures include:

- Alleviating anxiety and stress
- Reduction of smoking and beverages
- Withdrawal of adrenergic drugs
- Management of digitalis intoxication
- Treatment of congestive heart failure
- Management of myocardial ischemia.

Antiarrhythmic drugs may be used in symptomatic patients with organic heart disease and significant ventricular ectopy in whom correction of precipitating factors does not suffice.

Patients with structural cardiac abnormalities, such as left ventricular hypertrophy (LVH), hypertrophic obstructive cardiomyopathy (HOCM), dilated cardiomyopathy (DCMP) and arrhythmogenic right ventricular dysplasia (ARVD) would benefit more from antiarrhythmic drugs.

Beta-blockers like propranolol and metoprolol are the drugs of choice for treatment of VPCs associated with anxiety, physical exercise, mitral valve prolapse or thyrotoxicosis.

Lidocaine and amiodarone are the drugs of choice for VPCs after myocardial infarction, cardiac surgery or catheterization.

VPCs occurring within 24 hours of myocardial infarction carry a better prognosis and indicate reperfusion. VPCs that appear after 24 hours carry a worse prognosis and merit drug treatment.

When a patient of congestive heart failure on digitalis develops significant VPCs, it has to be decided on clinical grounds whether digitalis should be continued to manage the heart failure or withdrawn in view of drug intoxication.

If digitalis is to be withdrawn, the antiarrhythmic drug of choice for digitalis-induced VPCs is phenytoin sodium which should be used in conjunction with standard therapy of digitalis intoxication.

Antiarrhythmic drugs may be used for control of VPCs but before initiating treatment with these drugs, the following issues need to be addressed to:

- Inappropriate drug usage, when the cause and effect relationship of VPCs to fatal ventricular arrhythmias has not been established
- Aggravation of underlying cardiac abnormalities, such as bradycardia and left ventricular dysfunction
- Proarrhythmic effect of these drugs with increased likelihood of other tachyarrhythmias
- Potential systemic side-effects associated with long-term antiarrhythmic therapy.

PAUSES DURING RHYTHM

A pause during normal regular sinus rhythm is a brief period of electrical inactivity on the ECG graph between successive beats, due to delay in onset of the next scheduled beat. A pause produces a larger gap between two successive beats than that seen in other parts of the rhythm.

The causes of pauses are:
- Premature beats
- Sinoatrial block
- Atrioventricular block.

Pause After Premature Beat

A premature beat, whether supraventricular or ventricular, is followed by a pause that compensates for its prematurity. This is known as the compensatory pause.

In the case of a supraventricular premature beat, there is a momentary suppression of SA node automaticity so that the next sinus beat is somewhat delayed. This results in an incomplete compensatory pause, that is, the interval between the beat preceding and following the premature beat, is less than twice the RR interval between two successive sinus beats.

In the case of ventricular premature beat, one sinus beat after the premature beat fails to activate the already depolarized ventricles while the second sinus beat occurs as usual. This results in a complete compensatory pause, which fully compensates for the prematurity of the ectopic beat. In other words, the interval between the beat preceding and that following the premature beat is exactly twice the RR interval between two successive sinus beats.

Pause After Blocked Premature Beat

A very premature atrial ectopic beat may find the AV node refractory to ventricular conduction, having already been traversed by the preceding sinus beat. Therefore, it gets blocked in the AV node and fails to inscribe a QRS complex. Nevertheless, the ectopic P wave of the premature beat deforms the T wave of the preceding sinus beat and is followed by a pause.

This premature ectopic P wave is the key to the differentiation of a nonconducted atrial premature beat from a pause due to sinoatrial block or atrioventricular block.

Pause Due to Sinoatrial Block

Sinoatrial (SA) block refers to an interference with the propagation of an impulse from the sinus node to the surrounding atrial myocardium, resulting in a delay or omission of an atrial response.

There are three degrees of sinoatrial block:

- **1° SA block:** First-degree SA block cannot be diagnosed from the ECG as there are no dropped beats. Electrophysiological study reveals slow sinoatrial conduction.
- **2° SA block:** In second-degree SA block, there is intermittent dropping of one more beats. In fact, an entire

beat (P wave with QRS complex) is dropped as neither atrial nor ventricular activation occurs **(Fig. 15.1)**.

If every second beat is dropped, that is, in a period of time when there should be 2 beats but there is only one beat, it is called 2:1 SA block. If every third beat is dropped, that is, 2 beats occur in a period of time when there should be 3 beats, it is called 3:2 SA block.

- **3° SA block:** This is also known as complete SA block, sinus arrest or atrial standstill **(Fig. 15.2)**. In third-degree SA block, there is a prolonged period of electrical inactivity or asystole following which either an escape rhythm from a subsidiary pacemaker takes over or prolonged asystole results in cardiac arrest.

Second-degree SA block needs to be differentiated from two other conditions.

- A nonconducted atrial ectopic beat also results in a pause resembling SA block. However, the nonconducted ectopic beat inscribes a premature ectopic P wave that superimposes on the T wave of the preceding sinus beat.

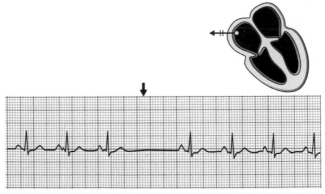

Fig. 15.1: Dropped beat due to second-degree sinoatrial block

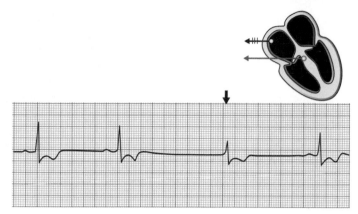

Fig. 15.2: Asystole followed by a junctional escape beat

- A second-degree atrioventricular block (AV block) also results in missing of a beat but in that case, the P wave is inscribed normally and only the QRS complex is missing.

Pause Due to Atrioventricular Block

Atrioventricular (AV) block refers to an interference with the propagation of an impulse from the atria to the ventricles, resulting in a delay or omission, of a ventricular response. There are three degrees of atrioventricular block:

- **1° AV block:** In first-degree AV block, there is only a delay in atrioventricular conduction of all beats. This is reflected in a prolonged PR interval in all beats, without any dropped beats **(Fig. 15.3)**
- **2° AV block:** In second-degree AV block, there is intermittent dropping of one or more beats. The P wave of the dropped beat is inscribed normally as atrial activation proceeds as usual. Only the QRS complex is missing because of failure of ventricular activation.

  Second-degree AV block is further classified as Mobitz Type I block and Mobitz Type II block.

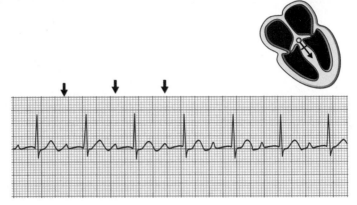

Fig. 15.3: First-degree AV block: Prolonged PR interval

In Mobitz Type I block, there is a gradual lengthening of the P-R interval from beat-to-beat till a P wave is not followed by a QRS complex **(Fig. 15.4)**, indicating a progressively increasing difficulty in AV nodal transmission. After the dropped beat the PR interval again shortens, indicating recovery of the AV node, but then begins to lengthen once again. This sequence of events is referred to as the Wenckebach phenomenon.

In Mobitz Type II block, the PR interval remains constant but there is intermittent dropping of beats, with some P waves not followed by a QRS complex **(Fig. 15.5)**. The ratio of the number of P waves to the number of QRS complexes represents the conduction sequence. If every second P wave is blocked, it is 2:1 AV block and if every third P wave is blocked, it is 3:2 AV block

- **3° AV block:** Third-degree AV block is also known as complete heart block. In this type of AV block, no sinus beat conducts to the ventricles as all of them get blocked in the AV node. Therefore, while the atria are activated by

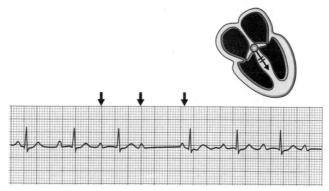

Fig. 15.4: Second-degree AV block (Mobitz Type I): Wenckebach phenomenon

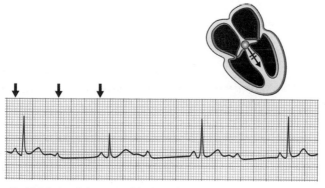

Fig. 15.5: Second-degree AV block (Mobitz Type II): 2:1 AV conduction

the SA node, the ventricles are activated by a subsidiary pacemaker in the His bundle system or in the ventricle. In other words, the atria and ventricles work independant of each other and asynchronously, leading to atrioventricular (AV) dissociation.

In third-degree AV block, P waves occur at a rate of 60–80 beats/minute that represents the discharge rate of the SA node. The rate of which QRS complexes occur depends upon the location of the subsidiary pacemaker.

If the lower pacemaker is situated in the His bundle system, the ventricular rate is 40–60 beats/minute and the QRS complexes are narrow since intraventricular conduction of beats is normal **(Fig. 15.6A)**.

However, if the lower pacemaker is situated in the ventricles, the rate is 20–40 beats/minute and the QRS complexes are wide as the ventricles are activated in a slow random fashion **(Fig. 15.6B)**.

Clinical Relevance of Pauses in Rhythm

Pause After Premature Beat

The compensatory pause after an atrial premature beat is incomplete while a ventricular premature beat is followed by a complete compensatory pause. This fact helps to differentiate a ventricular premature beat from an atrial premature beat conducted aberrantly to the ventricles.

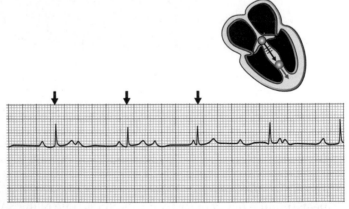

Fig. 15.6A: Third-degree (complete) AV block: Narrow QRS complexes

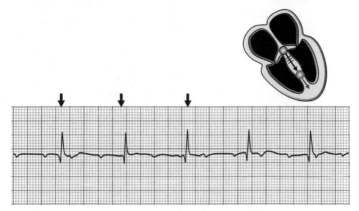

Fig. 15.6B: Third-degree (complete) AV block: Wide QRS complexes

An inordinately long pause after an atrial premature beat (prolonged sinus node recovery time) indicates sinus node dysfunction, the so called 'sick sinus syndrome'.

The awareness of a ventricular premature beat by the patient and its clinical recognition depend upon the compensatory pause and the increased force of the sinus beat following the premature beat.

Pause After Blocked Premature Beat

Atrial premature beat that fail to conduct to the ventricles produce pauses that resemble those due to SA block or AV block. Proper recognition of such pauses is important as their clinical significance and management are different.

Nonconducted atrial premature beats are frequently observed in elderly patients who have advanced AV nodal disease and in the presence of digitalis toxicity.

Pause Due to Second-Degree SA Block

Sinoatrial block may be observed in these conditions:
- Drugs, e.g. beta-blockers, diltiazem, digitalis
- Sinus node dysfunction or sick sinus syndrome.

The "sick sinus syndrome" is a clinical condition caused by a diseased sinus node which fails to produce sufficient impulses. It is observed in elderly patients and is believed to be caused by a degenerative condition (amyloidosis) or infiltration of the atria by a fibrocalcerous process.

The ECG features of sick sinus syndrome are:
- Sinus bradycardia
- Sinoatrial block
- Slow atrial fibrillation
- Junctional escape rhythm.

Other clinical features of this syndrome are:
- Inadequate tachycardia with stimuli
- Atropine resistant bradyarrhythmias
- Excessive beta-blocker sensitivity
- Alternating fast & slow rhythms (the 'brady-tachy' syndrome).

Symptoms of sick sinus syndrome are:
- Dizziness, syncope or fainting attacks
- Fatigue and dyspnea from heart failure
- Palpitations and angina pectoris
- Mental confusion and memory defects.

Treatment of sick sinus syndrome includes:
- Drugs to increase the heart rate, e.g. atropine and sympathomimetic drugs
- Pacemaker insertion if symptoms due to bradycardia are frequent and severe
- Antiarrhythmic drugs for tachyarrhythmias which can be used only if an artificial pacemaker is in place or else they may cause severe bradycardia.

Pause Due to Second-Degree AV Block

Atrioventricular block (second-degree) may be observed in the following conditions:
- Acute febrile illness
  - ➡ Rheumatic fever
  - ➡ Diphtheria.
- Drug therapy
  - ➡ Digitalis
  - ➡ Diltiazem
  - ➡ Beta-blockers.
- Coronary artery disease
  - ➡ Inferior wall infarction
  - ➡ Right coronary artery spasm.

The occurrence of AV block in a febrile illness like rheumatic fever or diphtheria indicates associated myocarditis. The fact that drugs like propranolol and diltiazem can cause AV block is put to use in the management of atrial tachycardia to reduce the ventricular rate.

Since the AV node receives its blood supply from the right coronary artery in 90% of subjects, transient AV blocks are observed in inferior wall myocardial infarction caused by occlusion of the right coronary artery. The same may occur when the right coronary artery undergoes spasm.

Mobitz Type I AV block is often acute in onset, runs a self-limited course, only occasionally produces symptoms, rarely progresses to complete AV block, carries a good prognosis and often requires no treatment.

Mobitz Type II AV block is often chronic, almost always pathological, likely to produce symptoms, such as dizziness and fainting, may progress to complete AV block, carries an adverse prognosis and often requires cardiac pacing.

In the management of symptomatic AV block, although drugs like atropine and adrenaline can temporarily accelerate the ventricular rate, cardiac pacing is the definitive form of treatment especially in patients with recurrent and severe symptoms.

Pauses Causing Bigeminal Rhythm

We have examined above the various causes of pauses during a regular rhythm. If these pauses occur regularly and are so timed that they follow a pair of beats, they produce a characteristic rhythm called bigeminal rhythm.

The causes of a bigeminal rhythm are:
- Alternate atrial premature beats (extrasystolic atrial bigeminy)
- Alternate ventricular premature beats (extrasystolic ventricular bigeminy)
- Blocked atrial ectopics after two beats
- 3:2 second-degree sinoatrial block
- 3:2 second-degree atrioventricular block.

Fast Regular Rhythm with Narrow QRS

REGULAR FAST RHYTHM

A regular cardiac rhythm that exceeds a rate of 100 beats per minute indicates rapid discharge of impulses from the pacemaker governing the rhythm of the heart.

If the QRS complexes during such a rhythm are narrow, it indicates normal intraventricular conduction and that the pacemaker is supraventricular in location, be it the SA node, the atrial myocardium or the AV junction.

Let us examine the specific arrhythmias that are associated with these features.

SINUS TACHYCARDIA

The occurrence of sinus node discharge at a rate exceeding 100 beats/minute constitutes sinus tachycardia. The rhythm is regular and the P wave as well as QRS morphology are obviously as in normal sinus rhythm **(Fig. 16.1)**.

Sinus tachycardia generally does not exceed a rate of 150 beats/minute as the AV node cannot conduct more than 150 impulses in a minute. Therefore, in sinus tachycardia, the RR interval ranges from 10 mm (heart rate 150) to 15 mm (heart rate 100).

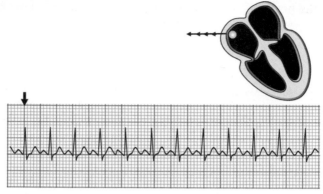

Fig. 16.1: Sinus tachycardia: Narrow QRS complexes; rate <150/minute

ATRIAL TACHYCARDIA

Atrial tachycardia or supraventricular tachycardia, is a fast regular rhythm produced by two possible mechanisms:

- Rapid impulse discharge from ectopic focus in the atrium (ectopic tachycardia; 10% cases)
- Repetitive circus movement in a closed reentrant circuit (reentrant tachycardia; 90% cases).

The circuit is either composed of two pathways within the AV node (AV nodal reentrant tachycardia—AVNRT; 50% cases) or consists of an AV nodal pathway and an accessory bypass tract alongside the AV node (AV reentrant tachycardia—AVRT; 40% cases). The two pathways of the reentrant circuit are connected to each other functionally, to form a closed loop.

An atrial impulse first passes anterogradely down one of the pathways, the other pathway being in the refractory period. The impulse then returns retrogradely through the other pathway, which has by now recovered its conductivity. In this way, repetitive circulation of impulses occurs to produce a sustained atrial tachycardia.

The heart rate in paroxysmal atrial tachycardia is 150–200 beats per minute **(Fig. 16.2)**, if a reentrant circuit is involved. It tends to be slower in ectopic atrial tachycardia (120–150 beats/min) as the AV node cannot conduct more than 150 atrial impulses per minute.

The heart rate can exceed a rate of 200 beats/minute if a true accessory bypass tract is involved as in the WPW syndrome. This is because in the WPW syndrome, the impulses can bypass the decremental influence of the AV node by passing down the accessory pathway.

In most cases of atrial tachycardia, the ventricular rate is the same as the atrial rate representing 1:1 AV conduction. This is always true for a reentrant tachycardia because the block of even a single impulse can interrupt the continuous reciprocating process and terminate the tachycardia. However, an ectopic atrial tachycardia can coexist with a physiological block, such as 2:1 AV block.

The contour and polarity of the P waves in atrial tachycardia is different from P wave morphology during sinus rhythm. In ectopic atrial tachycardia, the P waves are generally upright while they may be inverted in reciprocating tachycardia,

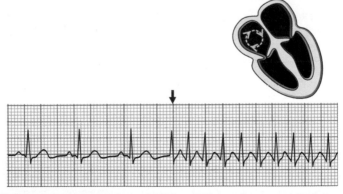

Fig. 16.2: AV reentrant tachycardia: Narrow QRS complexes, rate >150/minute

signifying retrograde atrial activation. The P waves are often not discernible in atrial tachycardia as they are fused with the T waves.

The QRS complex of an atrial tachycardia has a normal narrow configuration if atrial impulses pass anterogradely through the AV node (orthodromic tachycardia). The QRS complexes are wide if atrial beats pass through the bypass tract and retrogradely through the AV node (antidromic tachycardia). At times, the atrial impulses find one of the two bundle branches refractory to conduction and pass down only one bundle branch. This produces a bundle branch block like configuration of the QRS complexes and is known as aberrant ventricular conduction of an atrial tachycardia.

Other causes of wide QRS complexes during atrial tachycardia are preexisting conditions producing QRS abnormalities; such as true bundle branch block, intra-ventricular conduction defect or the WPW syndrome.

The differences between sinus tachycardia and atrial tachycardia have been tabulated in **Table 16.1**.

The features of a paroxysmal atrial tachycardia that differentiate it from sinus tachycardia are:

TABLE 16.1: Differences between sinus and atrial tachycardia

	Atrial tachycardia	*Sinus tachycardia*
Heart rate	150–220/minute	100–150/minute
Regularity	Clock-like	Respiratory variation
P wave	Ectopic/Inverted	Normal
Onset	Sudden onset	Gradual warm up
Effect of vagal maneuvers	Termination	Slowing of rate
ECG during normal rhythm	APCs or WPW syndrome	Often normal

TABLE 16.2: Differences between ectopic and reentrant tachycardia

	Ectopic tachycardia	*Reentrant tachycardia*
Heart rate	120–150/minute	More than 150/minute
Onset and offset	Gradual	Sudden
P wave	Ectopic. Visible	Inverted. Rarely visible
A-V block	Can coexist	Never. 1:1 conduction
Effect of vagal maneuvers	Slowing	Termination
Past history	Not significant	Of previous episodes
Heart disease	May be present	Generally absent

- Heart rate of 150–220 beats/minute
- Clock-like regularity of rhythm
- Sudden onset of tachycardia
- P waves different from sinus P waves
- History of recurrent episodes of tachycardia
- Abrupt termination with vagal maneuvers.

An atrial tachycardia arising from an ectopic focus can be differentiated from a tachycardia due to a reentrant mechanism by the features mentioned in **Table 16.2**.

An atrial tachycardia with aberrant ventricular condition closely resembles a ventricular tachycardia. Features that favor the diagnosis of atrial tachycardia are:

- Clock-like regular rhythm
- Maintained P-QRS relationship
- QRS width less than 0.14 second
- Stable hemodynamic parameters
- Termination with carotid sinus pressure.

ATRIAL FLUTTER

Atrial flutter is a fast rhythm caused by rapid discharge of an ectopic atrial focus or alternatively, a self-perpetuating re-entrant circuit located in the atrium. Therefore, it is obvious that atrial flutter is akin to atrial tachycardia.

The major difference between atrial flutter and atrial tachycardia is in terms of the atrial rate. The atrial rate in atrial flutter is 220–350 beats per minute. The P waves are replaced by flutter waves (F waves) that occur rapidly at this rate and give the baseline a corrugated or saw-toothed appearance **(Fig. 16.3)**.

It is understandable that all flutter waves cannot activate the ventricles. Therefore, there exists a physiological A-V block whereby the ventricular rate is a fraction of the atrial rate. If there is 2:1 physiological A-V block, two flutter waves are followed by one QRS complex while if the block is 4:1, four flutter waves are followed by one QRS complex.

Generally, the even ratios of physiological A-V block (2:1, 4:1) are more common than odd ratios (3:1, 5:1). Assuming an atrial flutter at an atrial rate of 300 beats/minute, with 2:1 block, the ventricular rate would be 150 beats/minute and with 4:1 block it would be 75 beats/minute.

Atrial flutter is quite akin to atrial tachycardia in terms of causation, mechanism and ECG features. The two conditions

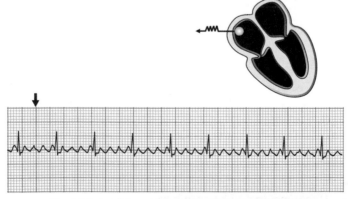

Fig. 16.3: Atrial flutter: Discrete F waves; regular rhythm

TABLE 16.3: Differences between atrial flutter and atrial tachycardia

	Atrial flutter	*Atrial tachycardia*
Atrial rate	220–350/minute	150–220/minute
Ventricular rate	1/2 or 1/4 of atrial rate (2:1 or 4:1 AV block)	Same as atrial rate (1:1 AV conduction)
P waves	Saw-tooth like flutter waves	Ectopic/inverted P waves
Effect of carotid sinus pressure	Increased degree of AV block	Termination in PAT. Slowing in ectopic tachycardia

can be differentiated from each other by the features enumerated in **Table 16.3**.

Atrial flutter with 2:1 physiological AV block resembles a sinus tachycardia at a rate of 120–150 beats/minute if one of the two flutter waves is buried in the QRS complex and the other is mistaken for the P wave. The diagnosis of atrial flutter can be clinched if after carotid sinus massage, AV nodal refractoriness increases and both the flutter waves become identifiable.

Clinical Relevance of Fast Regular Narrow QRS Rhythm

Sinus Tachycardia

Sinus tachycardia represents response of the SA node to a variety of physiological and pathological stimuli, mediated by the nervous and hormonal control over the pacemaker discharge rate.

The causes of sinus tachycardia are:
- Exercise and anxiety
- Fever and volume depletion
- Hypoxemia and anemia
- Hypotension and heart failure

- Thyrotoxicosis and pregnancy
- Caffeine and nicotine
- Atropine and beta-agonists
- Hemorrhage and hypoglycemia
- Pericarditis and myocarditis
- Massive pulmonary embolism.

In febrile patients, for each degree Fahrenheit rise in temperature, the heart rate rises by 8–10 beats/minute. A sinus tachycardia in excess of the predicted rate is a feature of myocarditis, rheumatic fever or bacterial endocarditis.

A sinus tachycardia at a rate less than expected in a febrile person is known as relative bradycardia and is observed in typhoid fever and in brucellosis.

Failure to develop sinus tachycardia in reponse to a physiological or pathological stimulus and in the absence of beta-blocker or calcium-blocker therapy is a sign of sinus node dysfunction, the so called sick sinus syndrome.

Sinus tachycardia is not a primary arrhythmia and therefore, treatment should be directed towards the basic underlying condition. Examples are antipyretics for fever, oxygen for hypoxemia, fluids for volume depletion and tranquilizers for emotional upset.

Specific therapy should be instituted when sinus tachycardia is an expression of the underlying disease. Such diseases include severe anemia, thyrotoxicosis, congestive heart failure, rheumatic fever and bacterial endocarditis.

Withdrawal of smoking, beverages, spices, anticholinergic drugs and adrenergic agents is mandatory to control the tachycardia. Propranolol and mild tranquilizers are indicated for supportive therapy of sinus tachycardia associated with anxiety, anemia and thyrotoxicosis.

Atrial Tachycardia

As a series of three or more successive atrial ectopic beats constitutes an atrial tachycardia, the causes of ectopic atrial tachycardia are similar to those of atrial premature beats. These include:

- Rheumatic fever
- Digitalis toxicity
- Thyrotoxicosis
- Myocardial ischemia
- Acute myocarditis
- Adrenergic drugs
- Cardiac surgery.

Paroxysmal reentrant atrial tachycardia is most often based on a reciprocal mechanism involving a bypass tract or dual intranodal pathway. Episodes of atrial tachycardia are one of the manifestations of pre-excitation syndrome, the WPW syndrome.

In the absence of WPW syndrome, paroxysmal atrial tachycardia (PAT) is generally not associated with organic heart disease. If properly managed, PAT does not alter life-expectancy and has an excellent prognosis.

PAT coexisting with the WPW syndrome carries a poorer prognosis because of the risk of degeneration into ventricular tachycardia.

A reentrant atrial tachycardia always exists with 1:1 AV conduction since the reciprocating circuit would break with the block of even a single beat. This is also the reason why vagal stimulation methods and drugs that block the A-V node can terminate the tachycardia.

On the other hand, an ectopic atrial tachycardia can coexist with AV block and is popularly known as 'PAT with block'. Digitalis toxicity is the most common cause of this rhythm.

Symptoms due to atrial tachycardia depend upon the atrial rate, the duration of the tachycardia and the presence of heart disease.

A fast atrial tachycardia causes palpitation and neck pulsations. Angina pectoris may occur due to increased myocardial oxygen demand and reduced coronary filling time.

Prolonged atrial tachycardia can cause dizziness or syncope due to decline in cardiac output (shortened ventricular filling time) and loss of atrial contribution to ventricular filling.

Termination of the tachycardia is often followed by polyuria due to the release of atrial natriuretic peptide (ANP) by myocardial stretch.

Atrial tachycardia needs to be differentiated clinically and electrocardiographically from various other rhythms that closely resemble it. Differentiation from sinus tachycardia is important since atrial tachycardia needs more aggressive treatment.

The causation and to some extent, the response to treatment of ectopic atrial tachycardia is somewhat different from that of reentrant tachycardia and they need to be differentiated from each other.

Since the heart rate in atrial tachycardia is rapid, P waves are not discernible and, therefore, differentiation from junctional tachycardia becomes difficult. However, since treatment of both is similar, the umbrella term supraventricular tachycardia (SVT) is used and further distinction becomes redundant.

Finally, atrial tachycardia with aberrant ventricular conduction needs to be identified as distinct from ventricular tachycardia since their causation, clinical presentation, prognosis and treatment are entirely different.

The Wolff-Parkinson-White (WPW) syndrome is a distinct electrocardiographic entity wherein an accessory pathway, the Bundle of Kent, connects the atrial to the ventricular myocardium, bypassing the AV node. This produces abnormalities of the QRS complex, PR interval, ST segment and the T wave, during sinus rhythm.

The clinical importance of the WPW syndrome lies in the fact that it predisposes to paroxysmal atrial tachycardia since the bypass tract forms a reentrant circuit with the regular conduction pathway. Paroxysmal tachycardia in the presence of WPW syndrome needs to be differentiated from a PAT without the accessory pathway since its management is somewhat different.

A paroxysm of atrial tachycardia in the presence of an underlying WPW syndrome is suggested if it meets one of the following criteria:

- ECG recorded in sinus rhythm shows a short PR interval, delta wave and a wide QRS complex
- The ventricular rate exceeds 200 beats/minute indicating absence of physiological AV block
- Inverted P waves are observed indicating retrograde atrial activation and conduction.

There are several modalities of treatment of PAT. Since reentry through an intranodal pathway or a bypass tract accounts for 90 percent of PAT, we shall first discuss the management of reentrant PAT.

The first step is to try methods of vagal stimulation so as to reduce AV conduction and consequently the ventricular rate. Vagal maneuvers that may be attempted include carotid sinus massage, supraorbital pressure, Valsalva maneuver or immersion of face in ice-cold water.

Carotid sinus massage is performed behind the angle of the mandible and over the carotid artery, for 5–10 seconds at a time. Before commencing massage, the carotid artery on both sides should be auscultated for a bruit. If a bruit is present, carotid massage should not be done or else an embolus may dislodge from an atheromatous plaque.

Carotid massage should be done on one side at a time and not simultaneously since bilateral massage can cause a precipitous fall in cerebral circulation.

If vagal maneuvers fail to abort the tachycardia, a drug acting on the AV node may be given intravenously.

The protocol of drug therapy for PAT is:

Adenosine 6 mg IV over 1–3 second; repeat 12 mg IV after 1–2 minute; repeat 12 mg IV after another 1–2 minute; till sinus rhythm is restored or 30 mg is given.

OR

Diltiazem 15–20 mg (0.25 mg/kg) IV over 2 minute; repeat 20–25 mg (0.35 mg/kg) IV over 2 minute after 15 minute if needed.

OR

Amiodarone 150 mg IV over 10 minute (15 mg/min); repeat 150 mg IV over 10 minute; repeat every 10 minute if needed.

Oral diltiazem, amiodarone or metoprolol is prescribed after restoration of sinus rhythm to prevent recurrence of PAT.

If a pacemaker is already in place, delivering a single programmed extrastimulus or overdrive pacing can break the reentrant circuit and restore sinus rhythm.

Electrical cardioversion with 80–100 Joules is the treatment of choice for atrial tachycardia associated with deranged hemodynamics and a low cardiac output.

Surgical ablation of the AV junction may be considered as a last resort in frequent, recurrent drug-refractory PAT which, however, makes the concomitant insertion of a permanent pacemaker mandatory.

The management of ectopic atrial tachycardia is similar to that of PAT with these differences:

- Vagal maneuvers are less likely to be effective
- Digoxin is to be avoided as it causes ectopic beats
- Programmed extra-stimulus cannot restore sinus rhythm
- Long-term prophylactic treatment is not indicated
- Electrical cardioversion and surgical ablation have no role.

The management of paroxysmal atrial tachycardia in the presence of WPW syndrome is also somewhat different.

- Vagal maneuvers would be useful only if anterograde conduction occurs through the AV node
- Digitalis is contraindicated as it enhances conduction down the accessory pathway and may precipitate ventricular fibrillation
- Diltiazem and metoprolol reduce tolerance to the high ventricular rate and precipitate congestive heart failure
- Amiodarone is the antiarrhythmic agent of choice for the long-term treatment and prevention of arrhythmias associated with the WPW syndrome.

Urgent electrical cardioversion is life-saving in atrial tachycardia associated with unstable hemodynamic parameters.

Cardioversion should be preceded by intravenous heparin and a transesophageal ECHO to exclude an atrial clot. It should follow-up by oral anticoagulation for 4 weeks.

The availability of sophisticated electrophysiological studies (EPS) to identify and locate bypass tracts and the development of ablative techniques have revolutionized the management of WPW syndrome.

For ablation of the bypass tract, high-frequency AC current is delivered through a thermistor-tipped catheter, which leads to localized heat coagulation.

Radiofrequency ablation (RFA) of the bypass tract can be offered to patients who report recurrent and frequent symptomatic episodes of PAT that produce hemodynamic compromise and are refractory to drug therapy.

RFA is the preferred form of treatment in these subsets:

- Very short PR interval on ECG
- Very short refractory period on EPS
- Familial syndrome and Ebstein anomaly
- High-risk professionals, e.g. aircraft pilots and military personnel.

Atrial Flutter

Atrial flutter is quite akin to ectopic tachycardia electrocardio-graphically, differing from it only in terms of the atrial rate. In terms of causation too, atrial flutter closely resembles atrial tachycardia.

Common causes are:
- Ischemic heart disease
- Rheumatic heart disease
- Acute respiratory failure
- Thyrotoxicosis
- Cor pulmonale
- Myocarditis
- Pericarditis
- Cardiac surgery.

Compared to its better known counterpart called atrial fibrillation, atrial flutter is less common and generally short-lived. It causes fewer symptoms and is less likely to cause a left atrial thrombus and subsequent risk of systemic embolization.

As far as the management of atrial flutter is concerned, the heart rate may be controlled by diltiazem or metoprolol as in atrial tachycardia. If conversion to sinus rhythm or to atrial fibrillation is the goal, digoxin or amiodarone may be used.

Digoxin converts atrial flutter to fibrillation with an increase in atrial rate. However, this is of advantage since the ventricular rate declines as the degree of concealed conduction increases. When digitalis is stopped, this often restores sinus rhythm.

If the patient's clinical status is unsatisfactory with angina, hypotension or heart failure, electrical cardioversion with a low energy shock of 10–50 Joules is the most effective form of treatment. In fact, atrial flutter is the most responsive of the tachyarrhythmias that revert with electrical cardioversion.

Normal Regular Rhythm with Narrow QRS

REGULAR NORMAL RHYTHM

A regular cardiac rhythm at a rate of 60–100 beats per minute is considered to be a normal rhythm.

If the QRS complexes during such a rhythm are narrow, it indicates normal intraventricular conduction and that the pacemaker is supraventricular in location. The pacemaker may be the SA node, in the atrial myocardium or at the AV junction.

Let us examine the specific arrhythmias that are associated with these features.

NORMAL SINUS RHYTHM

The occurrence of sinus node discharge at a rate of 60–100 beats/minute constitutes a normal sinus rhythm.

The rhythm is regular, the P wave and QRS complex are normal in morphology and they are related to each other with a 1:1 relationship.

ATRIAL TACHYCARDIA WITH 2:1 AV BLOCK

In atrial tachycardia, the atrial rate varies from 150 to 200 beats/minute. If all atrial impulses are conducted to the ventricles, the ventricular rate is identical.

However, if there exists a physiological 2:1 AV block and every alternate P wave is followed by a QRS complex, the ventricular rate is half of the atrial rate or 75–100 beats/minute.

Such a rhythm superficially resembles a normal sinus rhythm with the difference that the PP interval between successive P waves reflects an atrial rate of 150–200 beats/minute.

ATRIAL FLUTTER WITH 4:1 AV BLOCK

In atrial flutter, the atrial rate varies from 220 to 350 beats/minute. Since all atrial impulses cannot conduct to the ventricles at this rate, there exists a physiological AV block and the ventricular rate is a fraction of the atrial rate.

If the physiological block is 4:1 and every fourth flutter wave is followed by QRS complex, the ventricular rate is one-fourth of the atrial rate or 60–80 beats/minute.

Such a rhythm superficially resembles a normal sinus rhythm with the difference that the P waves are replaced by rapidly occurring flutter waves.

Atrial flutter can be differentiated from atrial tachycardia (atrial rate 150 to 200 beats/minute) with 2:1 block by the fact that the FF interval between successive F waves indicates an atrial rate of 220 to 350 beats/minute.

JUNCTIONAL TACHYCARDIA

Junctional tachycardia is an ectopic rhythm originating from a latent subsidiary pacemaker located in the AV junction. Normally, this pacemaker is subdued when the cardiac rhythm is governed by the SA node. However, when the junctional pacemaker undergoes enhancement of its inherent automaticity, it produces a junctional tachycardia.

This rhythm is also known as nonparoxysmal junctional tachycardia to differentiate it from extrasystolic junctional tachycardia produced by a series of three or more junctional premature beats. Nonparoxysmal junctional tachycardia is also known as accelerated junctional rhythm.

Junctional tachycardia produces a regular rhythm at a rate of 60–100 beats/minute which is greater than the inherent rate of the junctional pacemaker (40–60 beats/min). The QRS complexes are narrow as in normal sinus rhythm **(Fig. 17.1)**.

The distinctive feature of a junctional tachycardia is the typical relationship between P waves and QRS complexes. If the atria are activated retrogradely from the junctional pacemaker, the P waves are inverted and related to the QRS complexes. They may just precede, just follow or be buried in the QRS complexes because of near-simultaneous atrial and ventricular activation.

If the atria continue to be activated by the SA node, the P waves are upright and unrelated to the QRS complexes. In that case, the junctional pacemaker only activates the ventricles.

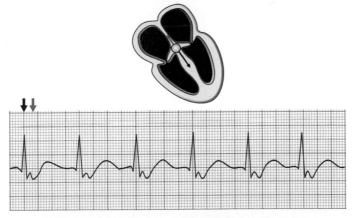

Fig. 17.1: Accelerated junctional rhythm: Inverted P waves just following QRS complexes

The ventricular rate is then slightly greater than the atrial rate, that is, the RR interval is slightly shorter than the PP interval.

Consequently, there is a progressive shortening of the PR interval in successive beats till the P wave merges in the QRS complex and then follows it. The P wave, so to say, marches through the QRS complex. This form of atrioventricular dissociation is called isorhythmic AV dissociation, since atrial and ventricular rates are nearly similar.

The P-QRS relationship mentioned above is typical of a rhythm originating from the AV junctional pacemaker. Inverted P waves just precede, just follow or are buried in the QRS complexes.

A junctional escape rhythm has similar features but occurs at a slower rate of 40 to 60 beats/minute which is the inherent rate of the junctional pacemaker.

An extrasystolic junctional tachycardia can be differentiated from accelerated junctional rhythm by the fact that it starts abruptly, is often paroxysmal in nature and the ventricular rate exceeds 120 beats/minute. The two conditions can be differentiated by features mentioned in **Table 17.1**.

Clinical Relevance of Regular Narrow QRS Rhythm

Normal Sinus Rhythm

A rhythm originating from the SA node at a rate of 60–100 beats/minute is a normal sinus cardiac rhythm. It is the most

TABLE 17.1: Junctional tachycardia versus junctional rhythm

	Extrasystolic junctional tachycardia	*Accelerated junctional rhythm*
Onset	Abrupt	Slow warm-up
Occurrence	Paroxysmal	Sustained
Ventricular rate	120–150/minute	60–100/minute

common, but by no means the only cause of a rhythm at this rate.

Atrial Tachycardia with AV Block

A fast atrial rhythm such as atrial tachycardia or atrial flutter, when associated with a fixed degree of physiological AV block, can also produce a normal ventricular rhythm at 60–100 beats/minute.

Junctional Tachycardia

A junctional tachycardia due to enhanced automaticity of the junctional pacemaker may be observed in:
- Digitalis toxicity
- Rheumatic carditis
- Inferior wall infarction
- Cardiac surgery
- Thyrotoxicosis.

When a febrile child develops a junctional tachycardia, rheumatic fever with carditis should be suspected. Thyrotoxicosis is a frequent cause of various atrial tachyarrhythmias, including junctional tachycardia.

In a coronary care unit, junctional tachycardia is often observed in cases of inferior wall myocardial infarction after they have recovered from AV block.

Open heart surgery, especially septal repair around the AV node, may be a cause of junctional tachycardia in the postoperative period.

If a patient is on digitalis for atrial fibrillation, regularization of the cardiac rhythm, even if sinus rhythm is not restored is often due to the onset of junctional tachycardia. This constitutes one of the markers of digitalis toxicity.

It is difficult and often futile to differentiate an extrasystolic junctional tachycardia from an ectopic tachycardia of atrial origin. They are both supraventricular tachycardias and similar in etiology, significance and management.

Junctional tachycardia is generally asymptomatic as it occurs at the same rate range as sinus rhythm. Moreover, its onset does not cause significant clinical deterioration as ventricular activation is normal. Only the loss of atrial contribution to ventricular filling (AV dissociation) can cause slight decline in cardiac output.

Active treatment of junctional tachycardia is generally not required as it is asymptomatic and has few hemodynamic consequences.

If treatment is required as in patients with poor cardiac reserve, management of the precipitating event is the first goal. This includes management of digitalis intoxication, treatment of rheumatic carditis and control of thyrotoxicosis.

If these do not suffice, atropine can be given to accelerate the sinus rate, overdrive the junctional rhythm and eliminate atrioventricular dissociation.

Antiarrhythmic drugs, electrical cardioversion and external pacing are unnecessary while vagal stimulation methods have no role in the management of junctional tachycardia.

Fast Irregular Rhythm with Narrow QRS

IRREGULAR FAST RHYTHM

A cardiac rhythm that exceeds a rate of 100 beats per minute indicates rapid discharge of impulses from the pacemaker governing the rhythm of the heart.

If the QRS complexes during such a rhythm are narrow, it indicates normal intraventricular conduction and that the pacemaker is supraventricular in location.

Further, if the rhythm is irregular, it signifies a variability either in impulse origin or in impulse conduction through the AV node.

Let us examine the specific arrhythmias that are associated with these features.

ATRIAL TACHYCARDIA WITH AV BLOCK

In atrial tachycardia, the atrial rate varies from 150 to 220 beats/minute. If all atrial impulses are conducted to the ventricles, the ventricular rate is identical.

However, if some atrial impulses are blocked in the AV node and this physiological AV block is variable, the QRS complexes occur at varying intervals to produce an irregular rhythm.

ATRIAL FLUTTER WITH AV BLOCK

In atrial flutter, the atrial rate varies from 220 to 350 beats/minute. Since all atrial impulses cannot conduct to the ventricles at this rate, there exists a physiological AV block and the ventricular rate is a fraction of the atrial rate.

Generally, the degree of AV block is fixed and occurs in even ratios such as 2:1, 4:1 and 8:1. If this physiological AV block is variable, the QRS complexes occur at varying intervals to produce an irregular rhythm.

MULTIFOCAL ATRIAL TACHYCARDIA

Ectopic atrial tachycardia is a fast rhythm produced by a rapid discharge of impulses from a single ectopic atrial focus. If impulses arise from numerous atrial foci, it constitutes a multifocal atrial tachycardia or a chaotic atrial rhythm.

Multifocal atrial tachycardia is a fast rhythm at a rate of 100– 150 beats/minute characte.ized by a beat-to-beat variability in P wave configuration representing a changing focus of origin of impulses **(Fig. 18.1)**.

It may not be possible to select the dominant P wave of sinus origin. The PR interval is also variable because of variability in AV conduction time, depending upon the focus of origin. Some P waves are premature, others are blocked and they vary in morphology from being upright to inverted.

The ventricular rhythm is irregular because of the varying degree of prematurity of atrial impulses and the occurrence of blocked atrial beats.

Multifocal atrial tachycardia needs to be differentiated from multiple atrial premature beats, occurring frequently during sinus rhythm. In the latter case, it is possible to select the dominant P waves of sinus origin. Moreover, the abnormal P waves occur prematurely, and the QRS complexes that succeed them are followed by compensatory pauses.

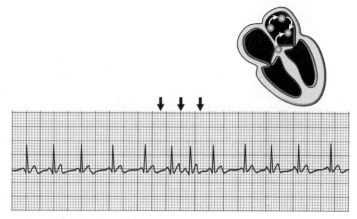

Fig. 18.1: Multifocal atrial tachycardia: Variable P waves

Multifocal atrial tachycardia (MAT) also closely resembles atrial fibrillation, since the ventricular rate is irregular in both rhythms. However, definite P waves are discernible in MAT while they are absent or replaced by fibrillatory waves (*f* waves) in atrial fibrillation.

A beat-to-beat variation in the P wave morphology is also a feature of a wandering pacemaker. However, in a wandering pacemaker rhythm, the heart rate is 60–100 beats/minute and not chaotic.

ATRIAL FIBRILLATION

Atrial fibrillation is a grossly irregular fast rhythm produced by the functional fractionation of the atria into numerous tissue islets. Therefore, instead of the sinus impulse spreading evenly and contiguously to all parts of atria, these islets are in various stages of excitation and recovery. Consequently, atrial activation is chaotic and ineffectual in causing hemodynamic pumping.

Although 400–500 fibrillatory impulses reach the AV node per minute, only 100–160 of them succeed in eliciting a ventricular response while others are blocked due to AV nodal refractoriness. The random activation of the ventricles produces a grossly irregular ventricular rhythm.

The hallmark of atrial fibrillation is absence of discrete P waves. Instead, there are numerous, small, irregular fibrillatory waves (*f* waves) that are difficult to identify individually but produce a ragged baseline (**Fig. 18.2**).

In long-standing atrial fibrillation, these undulations are minimal and produce a nearly flat baseline. As mentioned earlier, the ventricular rate is grossly irregular and varies from 100 to 160 beats per minute.

Atrial fibrillation can be differentiated from multifocal atrial tachycardia (MAT) by the fact that P waves are absent or replaced by fibrillatory waves, while definite P waves are discernible in MAT.

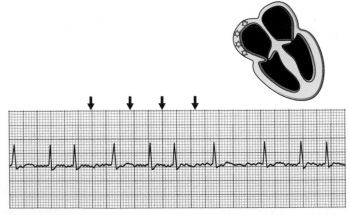

Fig. 18.2: Atrial fibrillation: Fine *f* waves; Irregular rhythm

TABLE 18.1: Differences between atrial flutter and atrial fibrillation

	Atrial flutter	*Atrial fibrillation*
Atrial rate	220–350 beats/minute	Over 350 beats/minute
Ventricular rate	Regular. Fraction of atrial rate	Variable. No relation to atrial rate
Atrial activity	Visible flutter (F) waves	Fine fibrillatory (f) waves
Baseline	Saw-toothed	Ragged
Ventricular activity	Constant RR interval	Variable RR interval

Atrial fibrillation can be differentiated from atrial flutter by the following features:
- Absence of P waves
- Irregular ventricular rate.

At times, precise differentiation between the two may be difficult and the rhythm is then known as "flutter-fibrillation", "coarse fibrillation" or "impure flutter". The differences between atrial flutter and atrial fibrillation are enlisted in **Table 18.1**.

Clinical Relevance of Fast Irregular Narrow QRS Rhythm

Atrial Tachycardia with Varying AV Block

The occurrence of a fast rhythm such as atrial tachycardia or atrial flutter with a variable interval between QRS complexes indicates a variability in conduction of the atrial impulses through the AV node.

Only an ectopic atrial tachycardia and not reentrant atrial tachycardia can coexist with AV block. Paroxysmal atrial tachycardia with AV block (PAT with block) is a popular term for this condition and digitalis toxicity is the most common cause of this rhythm.

Multifocal Atrial Tachycardia

The most frequent cause (in 80–90% cases) of multifocal atrial tachycardia is chronic obstructive lung disease with cor pulmonale and respiratory failure in a seriously ill elderly patient.

Aggravating factors that often coexist are:

- Respiratory tract infection
- Theophylline or digitalis
- Coronary artery disease
- Hypoxia and hypercapnia
- Electrolyte imbalance
- Alcohol intoxication.

Multifocal atrial tachycardia not only mimics, but often heralds the onset of atrial fibrillation. It has serious prognostic implications and carries a high mortality rate.

The treatment of aggravating factors and improvement of the pulmonary condition are the most important principles in the management of multifocal atrial tachycardia.

Necessary measures include treatment of infection with antibiotics, withdrawal of offending drugs, correcting electrolyte imbalance and administering oxygen.

Multifocal atrial tachycardia is not only refractory to antiarrhythmic drugs like verapamil, beta-blockers and digitalis, but these can worsen the cardiorespiratory status and are hence to be avoided.

Atrial Fibrillation

Atrial fibrillation may be observed in virtually all forms of organic heart disease. Causes of atrial fibrillation are:

- Persistent atrial fibrillation (>7 days)
  - ➡ Congenital heart disease (ASD)
  - ➡ Rheumatic heart disease (MS)
  - ➡ Coronary artery disease (MR)

➤ Hypertensive heart disease
➤ Idiopathic cardiomyopathy
➤ Cardiac trauma or surgery
➤ Constrictive pericarditis.
- Paroxysmal atrial fibrillation (<7 days)
  ➤ Acute alcoholic intoxication
  ➤ Recurrent pulmonary embolism
  ➤ Thyrotoxicosis
  ➤ WPW syndrome
  ➤ Sick sinus syndrome
  ➤ Lone atrial fibrillation.

In atrial fibrillation, the ventricular rate generally varies from 100 to 150 beats per minute. Faster rates are observed in children, patients of thyrotoxicosis and in the presence of WPW syndrome.

Slower rates are observed during drug treatment with propranolol/atenolol or verapamil/diltiazem as these drugs block the AV node. Elderly patients with AV nodal disease may also manifest slow atrial fibrillation.

Regularization of the ventricular rate in a patient on digitalis for atrial fibrillation indicates the onset of junctional tachycardia and is a manifestation of digitalis toxicity.

Symptoms due to atrial fibrillation depend upon:
- The ventricular rate
- The severity of heart disease
- The effectiveness of treatment.

The symptoms frequently observed in atrial fibrillation along with their causation are:
- Palpitations (fast heart rate)
- Angina (increased myocardial oxygen demand and shortened coronary filling time)
- Fatigue (low cardiac output due to loss of atrial contribution to ventricular filling)
- Dyspnea (pulmonary congestion due to ineffectual atrial contraction)

- Regional ischemia (systemic embolization from atrial thrombus).

Atrial fibrillation may be life-threatening in these situations:

- Low cardiac output state with pulmonary edema due to left ventricular dysfunction
- Non-compliant ventricle when atrial contribution to ventricular filling is crucial
- WPW syndrome where conduction of impulses down the accessory pathway can precipitate ventricular tachycardia or fibrillation
- Injudicious treatment of atrial fibrillation such as digitalis usage in WPW syndrome and diltiazem or propranolol for sick sinus syndrome.

Clinical signs of atrial fibrillation are:

- *Pulse:* Irregular and fast pulse rate; pulse deficit, which is radial pulse rate less than the heart rate counted by cardiac auscultation
- *BP:* Low systolic blood pressure; variable pulse pressure
- *JVP:* Raised jugular venous pressure; absent '*a*' waves
- *Heart sounds:* Beat-to-beat variability in the intensity of the first heart sound.

Various modalities of treatment are available for the management of atrial fibrillation, the judicious use of which can result in clinical improvement of most patients.

- *Antiarrhythmic drugs:* If hemodynamics of the patient are stable, it suffices to control the ventricular rate by a drug that prolongs the refractory period of the AV node.

Diltiazem, esmolol or amiodarone may be administered intravenously to control the heart rate.

Diltiazem 15–20 mg over 2 minute; repeat after 15 minute.

Esmolol 500 µg/kg over 1–2 minute; repeat after 10–15 minute.

Amiodarone 150 mg over 10 minute; repeat after 10 minute.

Oral diltiazem, amiodarone or metoprolol can be prescribed for long-term rate control but should be avoided in the presence of heart failure, in which case digoxin is preferable.

These drugs are contraindicated in the presence of WPW syndrome where AV nodal block would increase the conduction of impulses down the accessory pathway and hence, the likelihood of ventricular fibrillation.

Amiodarone is very effective in the prevention of paroxysmal atrial fibrillation. Moreover, it is effective and safe in the presence of the WPW syndrome as it suppresses conduction of impulses down the accessory pathway.

If rate control does not suffice and symptoms persist, pharmacological cardioversion to restore sinus rhythm may be tried. Drugs used for this indication are dronedarone, flecainide, propafenone, sotalol and ibutilide. Limitations of this approach are modest efficacy, adverse effects, high recurrence rate and proarrhythmic potential.

- *Anticoagulants:* Long-standing atrial fibrillation produces stasis of blood in the left atrium and promotes the development of thrombi in the atrial cavity and atrial appendage.

  Dislodged fragments of these thrombi can enter the systemic circulation as emboli and settle down in any arterial territory to produce effects of regional ischemia.

  Examples are blindness due to retinal artery occlusion, hemiparesis due to cerebral circulation, impairment and ischemia of a limb due to brachioradial or ileofemoral obstruction.

  Anticoagulants such as coumarin and warfarin are required for long-term use in chronic atrial fibrillation to reduce likelihood of systemic embolization. This particularly applies to patients of rheumatic heart disease and prosthetic valve recipients as well as those with previous history of thromboembolism (stroke, TIA) and documented cardiac thrombus.

Anticoagulation is also indicated two weeks before and several weeks after electrical cardioversion since restoration of sinus rhythm and atrial function is likely to expel systemic emboli.

- *Electrical defibrillation:* If the patient's clinical status is poor and hemodynamics are unstable, electrical cardioversion with 100–200 Joules energy is the treatment of choice in an attempt to restore sinus rhythm.

  There are two requisites before cardioversion is attempted. Firstly, the patient should not have received digitalis in the previous 48 hours. Digitalis not only increases the threshold for defibrillation but also predisposes to the risk of life-threatening arrhythmias. Secondly, anticoagulation should be initiated before cardioversion and continued for at least 4 weeks later. This is because atrial thrombi are likely to dislodge as emboli, once sinus rhythm is restored. Cardioversion should not be attempted, if there is a documented left atrial clot.

  It is difficult to restore sinus rhythm with cardioversion, if atrial fibrillation is of more than one year duration and the left atrium is enlarged beyond 4.5 cm in diameter.

- *Radiofrequency ablation (RFA):* When all conventional remedies have been exhausted and a number of investigational agents have failed to treat atrial fibrillation, a final option is of RFA.

  Suitable candidates for RFA are those with significant symptoms who are refractory or intolerant to several antiarrhythmic agents.

  Prerequisites are age below 70 years, left atrial size less than 5 cm and absence of obesity or heart failure.

  Advantage is not only freedom from symptoms, but also from toxic effects of antiarrhythmic agents and the need to monitor anticoagulant therapy.

19

Fast Regular Rhythm with Wide QRS

FAST WIDE QRS RHYTHM

A regular cardiac rhythm that exceeds a rate of 100 beats per minute indicates rapid discharge of impulses from the pacemaker governing the rhythm of the heart.

If the QRS complexes during such a rhythm are wide, three possibilities have to be considered:

- The rhythm is ventricular in origin in which case ventricular activation is through myocardium and not the specialized conduction system
- The rhythm is supraventricular in origin but impulses are conducted aberrantly to the ventricles through one of the two branches of the His bundle
- The rhythm is supraventricular in origin but there are preexisting wide QRS complexes.

Let us go into the individual features of these rhythms.

VENTRICULAR TACHYCARDIA

Ventricular tachycardia is a fast regular rhythm produced by two possible mechanisms:

- Enhanced automaticity of a latent ventricular pacemaker producing rapid discharge of impulses.
- Repetitive circus movement of an impulse in a closed re-entrant circuit around a fixed anatomical substrate in the ventricular myocardium.

Ventricular tachycardia may be sustained (lasting >30 second) or nonsustained (lasting <30 second). It may be monomorphic (similar QRS complexes) or polymorphic (variable QRS complexes).

The heart rate in ventricular tachycardia is generally 150 to 200 beats per minute. The rhythm is usually slightly irregular in contrast to the perfect regularity of an atrial tachycardia. The QRS complexes are bizarre and wide, exceeding 0.14 second in width and do not conform to a bundle branch block pattern **(Fig. 19.1)**.

The atria may continue to be activated by the S-A node, but the P-waves are generally not visible as they are buried in the wide QRS complexes.

During ventricular tachycardia, the QRS pattern in all precordial leads is similar (concordant pattern) and the R/S ratio in lead V_6 is less than 1. Moreover, there is left axis deviation or a north-west QRS axis.

A ventricular tachycardia closely resembles an atrial tachycardia that is conducted aberrantly to the ventricles.

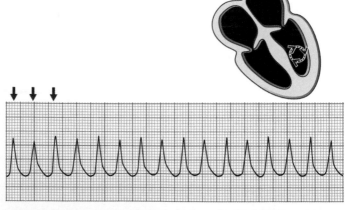

Fig. 19.1: Monomorphic ventricular tachycardia: Similar QRS complexes

Features that favor the diagnosis of ventricular tachycardia are:

- Slight irregularity of rhythm
- Lack of P-QRS relationship
- QRS width >0.14 second with bizarre shape
- Compromised hemodynamic parameters
- Presence of serious organic heart disease
- No response to carotid sinus pressure.

A peculiar variety of ventricular tachycardia called polymorphic ventricular tachycardia is characterized by phasic variation of the QRS complex amplitude and direction **(Fig. 19.2)**. Polymorphic VT is often associated with a prolonged QT interval and rarely with a normal QT interval.

A series of ventricular complexes are up-pointing and then down-pointing. This phenomena occurs in a repetitive continuum.

Since this sometimes gives the appearance of rotation of QRS complexes around the isoelectric line, it is designated

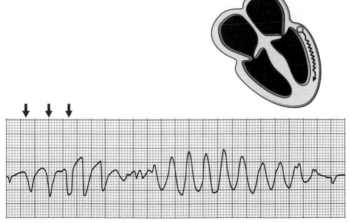

Fig. 19.2: Polymorphic ventricular tachycardia: Changing QRS configuration

as torsades de pointes, a ballet term which literally means "twisting of points".

Torsade de pointes is, as a rule, associated with prolongation of the QT interval. The prolonged QT interval favors the occurrence of a ventricular premature beat that coincides with the T-wave of the preceding beat (R-on-T phenomenon) and initiates the ventricular tachycardia.

SUPRAVENTRICULAR TACHYCARDIA WITH ABERRANT VENTRICULAR CONDUCTION

Most often, a supraventricular tachycardia is characterized by narrow QRS complexes as a result of synchronized ventricular activation through the specialized conduction system.

Occasionally, the supraventricular impulses find one of the two bundle branches refractory to conduction. In that case, the impulses are conducted only through the other bundle branch producing a situation of aberrant ventricular conduction. Understandably, the QRS complexes conform to a bundle branch block pattern.

The differences between ventricular tachycardia and supraventricular tachycardia with aberrant ventricular conduction are given in **Table 19.1**.

Essentially, the hallmark of ventricular tachycardia is evidence of dissociation between the atria and the ventricles.

The intensity of the first heart sound (S_1) is variable because of variability of the ventricular filling time. Cannon '*a*' waves are seen in the neck veins because of atrial contraction on a closed tricuspid valve.

Capture beats and fusion beats are produced by an atrial stimulus, occasionally finding the ventricular conduction system receptive to depolarization. A capture beat "captures" the ventricle completely to produce a normal narrow QRS complex in the midst of a ventricular tachycardia.

TABLE 19.1: Differences between ventricular tachycardia and SVT with aberrant conduction

	Ventricular tachycardia	*SVT with aberrancy*
Regularity of rhythm	Slightly irregular	Clocklike
P-QRS relationship	AV dissociation	Maintained
Heart sounds	Variable S_1	Constant S_1
Cannon waves	May be seen	Never seen
Capture/fusion beats	May be seen	Never seen
QRS width	>0.14 second	0.12–0.14 second
QRS morphology	Bizarre	Triphasic
QRS V_1–V_6	rS V_1–V_6	rS–Rs
R–R' height	R > R'	R' > R
QRS axis	Leftward	Normal
Hemodynamics	Compromised	Stable
Organic heart disease	Often present	Often absent
Response to carotid sinus massage	No response elicited	Slowing or termination

A fusion beat "captures" the ventricle partially to produce a QRS complex, which is a blend of normal narrow QRS and a VPC-like QRS complex.

SUPRAVENTRICULAR TACHYCARDIA WITH PREEXISTING QRS ABNORMALITY

It is known that certain conditions produce an abnormality of ventricular conduction even in normal sinus rhythm, causing an abnormality of QRS morphology.

Three well-known examples are:
- Bundle branch block
- WPW syndrome
- Intraventricular conduction defect.

If a supraventricular tachycardia occurs in the presence of a preexisting QRS abnormality, it is naturally expected to have wide QRS complexes.

A bundle branch block produces a triphasic QRS contour while an intraventricular conduction defect results in bizarre QRS morphology. The WPW syndrome is characterized by a delta wave on the ascending limb of the QRS complex.

Clinical Relevance of Fast Regular Wide QRS Rhythm

Ventricular Tachycardia

A series of three or more successive ventricular ectopic beats constitutes a ventricular tachycardia.

A ventricular tachycardia that lasts for more than 30 seconds and requires cardioversion for termination is called sustained ventricular tachycardia. A nonsustained ventricular tachycardia lasts for less than 30 seconds and ends spontaneously.

Ventricular tachycardia is considered repetitive or recurrent, if three or more discrete episodes are documented, while chronic ventricular tachycardia is that in which recurrent episodes occur for over a month.

As three or more ventricular premature complexes (VPCs) constitute ventricular tachycardia (VT), the causes of VT are similar to those of VPCs.

Causes of nonsustained ventricular tachycardia are:
- Pharmacological agents
  - ⇢ Theophylline
  - ⇢ Sympathomimetics
- Acute myocardial insult
  - ⇢ Ischemia
  - ⇢ Reperfusion

- Metabolic disorder
  - ⟶ Hypoxia
  - ⟶ Acidosis
  - ⟶ Hypokalemia
- Cardiac trauma
  - ⟶ Surgical
  - ⟶ Accidental
  - ⟶ Catheterization
- Drug intoxication
  - ⟶ Digitalis
  - ⟶ Quinidine.

Sustained ventricular tachycardia (scar VT) is more often based on structural heart disease where a fixed anatomical substrate facilitates a reentrant mechanism.

Causes of sustained ventricular tachycardia are:

- Myocardial scar
  - ⟶ Infarction
  - ⟶ Aneurysm
- Myocardial disease
  - ⟶ Cardiomyopathy
  - ⟶ Myocarditis
  - ⟶ RV dysplasia
- Congestive failure
  - ⟶ Ischemic
  - ⟶ Hypertensive
- Valvular abnormality
  - ⟶ Rheumatic heart disease
  - ⟶ Mitral valve prolapse.

Symptoms due to ventricular tachycardia depend on:

- The ventricular rate
- The duration of tachycardia
- Presence or absence of heart disease
- Severity of heart disease, if it is present.

Symptoms of sustained ventricular tachycardia with underlying heart disease and their causation are:

- Palpitation (fast heart rate)
- Angina (increased oxygen demand and shortened coronary filling time)
- Dyspnea (pulmonary edema due to loss of atrial contribution to ventricular filling)
- Syncope (low cardiac output state).

Clinical signs often observed during sustained ventricular tachycardia are:

- *Pulse:* Fast and irregular pulse
- *BP:* Low systolic blood pressure
- *JVP:* Raised jugular venous pressure
- *Heart sounds:* Systolic murmur and S_3 gallop.

The prognosis of sustained ventricular tachycardia depends upon the seriousness of the underlying cardiac disease, particularly severity of coronary disease and degree of left ventricular dysfunction. The prognosis is particularly poor in ventricular tachycardia developing after acute myocardial infarction.

Markers of electrical instability in survivors of acute myocardial infarction are:

- Documented serious ventricular arrhythmias on 24 hour ambulatory Holter monitoring or detected by an implantable loop recorder (ILR)
- Reproducible sustained ventricular tachycardia on programed electrical stimulation (PES)
- Late depolarization potentials detected on signal averaged electrocardiogram (SAECG)
- Q-T dispersion and T wave alternans.

The management of ventricular tachycardia depends upon the following factors:

- Sustained/nonsustained tachycardia
- Symptomatic/asymptomatic tachycardia

- Presence/absence of heart disease
- Presence/absence of cardiac decompensation.

The modalities of treatment of ventricular tachycardia are pharmacological, electrical and surgical.

- **Pharmacological therapy:** Nonsustained ventricular tachycardia in an asymptomatic individual without organic heart disease only requires withdrawal of sympathomimetic drugs, and correction of any metabolic disorder or electrolyte imbalance.

  If the ventricular tachycardia is sustained and symptomatic, sympathetic stimulation by stress, exercise or adrenergic drugs is the most common cause, in the absence of heart disease. This is known as catecholaminergic VT. Such patients respond well to beta-blockade with metoprolol.

  Polymorphic VT with normal Q-T interval is observed in myocardial ischemia, infarction, myocarditis and arrhythmogenic right ventricular dysplasia (ARVD). Such patients too respond well to beta-blockers.

  If sustained symptomatic ventricular tachycardia occurs in the presence of organic heart disease, the line of treatment depends upon the hemodynamic status. All such patients are best managed in an intensive cardiac care unit under the expert guidance of a cardiologist.

  If the hemodynamics are stable, pharmacological anti-arrhythmic therapy is initiated (chemical cardioversion). The drugs of choice are lidocaine and amiodarone. First, a bolus dose of the drug is administered intravenously, to be followed by a maintenance infusion

  The protocol of IV drug therapy of VT is:

  Amiodarone 150 mg IV over 10 minute (15 mg/min): Repeat 150 mg IV every 10 minute as needed.

  OR

  Lidocaine 0.5–0.75 mg/kg IV; repeat 0.5–0.75 mg/kg IV every 5–10 minute as needed to a maximum of 3 mg/kg.

Once sinus rhythm is restored, an infusion of the rhythm converting drug is initiated as:

Amiodarone 360 mg IV over next 6 hrs (1 mg/min); maintain at 540 mg IV over next 18 hours (0.5 mg/min)

OR

Lidocaine 2–4 mg/min (30–60 µg/kg/min).

Once the crisis period has been tided over, oral maintenance treatment with amiodarone may be instituted to prevent recurrence. Alternative drugs are flecainide, ibutilide, propafenone and sotalol.

Although one of these drugs may be used empirically, the ideal method is to select one of these drugs after an electrophysiological study.

The drug that renders the ventricular tachycardia noninducible by programed electrical stimulation, is the one most likely to prevent recurrence of ventricular tachycardia.

- **Electrical cardioversion:** If the hemodynamics are compromised with hypotension, myocardial ischemia, congestive heart failure and cerebral hypoperfusion, the ventricular tachycardia needs prompt termination by cardioversion.

  A nonsynchronized electrical shock of 50–100 J is the procedure of choice. It may be repeated with increasing energy of shock till sinus rhythm is restored. If to begin with, there is circulatory collapse and the peripheral pulses are not palpable, the initial dose of the DC shock should be 200–360 J.

  Once sinus rhythm has been restored, long-term oral pharmacological treatment may be initiated.

- **Surgical treatment:** Since a fixed anatomic substrate such as myocardial scar from previous infarction is often the basis of recurrent ventricular tachycardia, a surgical procedure can be offered for permanent cure.

Surgical techniques available are endocardial resection and encircling ventriculotomy

The modalities of treating polymorphic VT with QT prolongation are quite different from those employed for monomorphic VT

- In the acute setting, drug therapy which is useful is the infusion of magnesium sulphate or isoproterenol (beta-blocker). If the patient responds to beta-blockade, long-term antiadrenergic therapy is initiated or cervical sympathetic ganglionectomy is offered
- If the patient does not respond to the above measures, overdrive ventricular pacing can be attempted. Alternatively electrical cardioversion is performed, particularly in the presence of ischemia, heart failure or hypotension
- An implantable cardioverter defibrillator (ICD) device is offered to those with history of recurrent syncope, family history of sudden cardiac death (SCD) or to survivors of cardiac arrest and nonresponders to beta-blocker therapy.

Normal Regular Rhythm with Wide QRS

NORMAL WIDE QRS RHYTHM

A regular cardiac rhythm at a rate of 60–100 beats per minute is considered to be a normal rhythm. If the QRS complexes during such a rhythm are wide, it indicates abnormal intraventricular conduction of the impulses from the SA node. The P waves and the QRS complexes during sinus rhythm maintain a 1:1 relationship with each other.

The well-known causes of wide QRS complexes during sinus rhythm are bundle branch block, intraventricular conduction defect and Wolff-Parkinson-White (WPW) syndrome. There is one more condition where wide QRS complexes arise from a ventricular pacemaker at a rate of 60–100 beats/minute and is known as accelerated idioventricular rhythm (AIVR).

Let us see how this rhythm differs from sinus rhythm with wide QRS complexes.

ACCELERATED IDIOVENTRICULAR RHYTHM

Accelerated idioventricular rhythm (AIVR) is an ectopic rhythm originating from a latent subsidiary pacemaker located in the ventricular myocardium. Normally, such a pacemaker is subdued when the cardiac rhythm is governed by the SA node.

However, when a ventricular pacemaker undergoes enhancement of its inherent automaticity, it produces an idioventricular rhythm. Since the heart rate during such rhythm exceeds the inherent ventricular rate, it is known as accelerated idioventricular rhythm (AIVR).

AIVR produces a regular rhythm at a rate of 60–100 beats/minute that is greater than the inherent rate of the ventricular pacemaker which is 20–40 beats/minute. The QRS complexes are bizarre and wide because of ventricular origin of the rhythm **(Fig. 20.1)**.

The distinctive feature of AIVR is atrioventricular dissociation or lack of relationship between the P waves and the QRS complexes. This is because, the ventricles are activated by the ventricular pacemaker, and the atria continue to be activated by the SA node.

AIVR can be differentiated from ventricular tachycardia only by the ventricular rate. The rate is 60–100 beats/minute

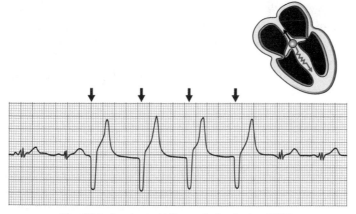

Fig. 20.1: Accelerated idioventricular rhythm (AIVR): Slow rhythm; Wide QRS complexes

in AIVR and 150–200 beats/minute in VT, although both rhythms originate from the ventricles.

Clinical Relevance of Regular Wide QRS Rhythm

Sinus Rhythm with Wide QRS Complexes

A normal sinus rhythm when associated with a conduction abnormality in the ventricles, produces wide QRS complexes. The morphology of the QRS complex depends upon the cause of the conduction abnormality. Importantly, the 1:1 P-QRS relationship is maintained during sinus rhythm.

The significance of wide QRS complexes during sinus rhythm depends upon the cause of QRS widening. Causes of wide QRS complexes are:

- Complete bundle branch block
- Intraventricular conduction defect
- Ventricular pre-excitation syndrome.

Accelerated Idioventricular Rhythm

AIVR is most often observed in coronary care units in a setting of acute myocardial infarction. It either occurs spontaneously or as a reperfusion arrhythmia after thrombolytic therapy. Other infrequent causes of AIVR are:

- Digitalis toxicity
- Rheumatic carditis
- Cardiac surgery.

The above causes of AIVR are quite akin to those of a junctional tachycardia or accelerated idiojunctional rhythm. Both are examples of an idiofocal tachycardia.

AIVR is most often picked up from the monitor screen of an intensive coronary care unit (ICCU). It needs to be differentiated from its more serious counterpart, ventricular tachycardia that often produces hemodynamic embarrassment, carries a poor prognosis and requires aggressive management. AIVR differs from VT, only in terms of the ventricular rate.

AIVR also needs to be differentiated from bundle branch block of recent onset, which is not uncommon in an ICCU setting. While AIVR produces bizarre and wide QRS complexes unrelated to P waves, bundle branch block is associated with a triphasic QRS contour and a maintained P-QRS relationship.

AIVR is usually asymptomatic as it occurs at the same rate range as sinus rhythm. It rarely causes serious hemodynamic embarrassment. Only the loss of atrial contribution to ventricular filling (AV dissociation) causes slight fall in cardiac output.

AIVR is usually transient and does not herald the onset of serious ventricular arrhythmias. Therefore, it is considered to be a benign arrhythmia with an excellent prognosis.

Active treatment of AIVR is generally not required as it is transient, asymptomatic and has few hemodynamic consequences. The hallmark of management of AIVR is constant observation. If treatment is required, it is only in patients with poor left ventricular function.

Atropine can be administered to accelerate the sinus rate, overdrive the ventricular rhythm and eliminate atrioventricular dissociation. Antiarrhythmic drugs, DC cardioversion and artificial pacing are unnecessary in the management of accelerated idioventricular rhythm.

Fast Irregular Rhythm with Bizarre QRS

IRREGULAR WIDE QRS RHYTHM

A cardiac rhythm that exceeds a rate of 100 beats per minute indicates a rapid discharge of impulses from the pacemaker governing the rhythm of the heart.

If the QRS complexes during such a rhythm are wide, bizarre looking and occur irregularly, it indicates a grossly abnormal pattern of intraventricular conduction and that the pacemaker is located in the ventricular myocardium.

Let us examine the specific arrhythmias that are associated with these features.

VENTRICULAR FLUTTER

Ventricular flutter is a fast ventricular rhythm produced either due to rapid discharge of impulses from a ventricular pacemaker or repetitive circus movement of an impulse in a reentrant circuit. Therefore, ventricular flutter is quite akin to ventricular tachycardia in terms of its mechanism.

The heart rate in ventricular flutter is 250–350 beats per minute and is irregular. The QRS complexes are very wide and bizarre in morphology while the P waves and T waves are not discernible **(Fig. 21.1)**.

In fact, merging of QRS complexes and T deflections produces a sine waveform. This is the differentiating feature

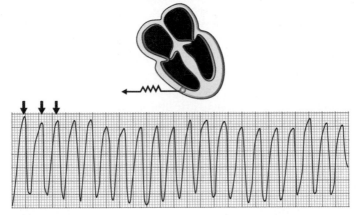

Fig. 21.1: Ventricular flutter: Undulating large waves; no QRS-T distinction

from ventricular tachycardia where QRS complexes and T waves are identifiable separately.

The deflections in ventricular flutter although wide and bizarre, they are large, constant in morphology and occur with slight irregularity. On the other hand, the deflections in ventricular fibrillation are relatively small, grossly variable in shape, height and width occurring in a totally chaotic fashion.

VENTRICULAR FIBRILLATION

Ventricular fibrillation is a grossly irregular rapid ventricular rhythm produced by a series of incoordinated and chaotic ventricular depolarizations at a rate of more than 350 beats per minute.

Instead of the ventricles being activated systematically through the conduction system to produce coordinated pumping, the ventricular myocardium is functionally fractionated into numerous tissue islets in various stages of excitation and recovery. Ventricular depolarization is thus chaotic and ineffectual in producing hemodynamic pumping.

Ventricular fibrillation manifests with rapidly and irregularly occurring small deformed deflections that are grossly variable in shape, height and width. The regular waveforms of P waves, QRS complexes and T waves cannot be identified and the isoelectric line seems to waver unevenly (**Fig. 21.2**).

Ventricular fibrillation can be differentiated from ventricular flutter by the fact that in the latter condition, although the QRS complexes are bizarre and wide, they are relatively large, constant in morphology and occur only with slight irregularity.

Ventricular fibrillation needs to be differentiated from complete cardiac arrest or asystole in which no ECG deflections are recorded. This is possible by the fact that no matter how small, some definite deflections are always recorded in ventricular fibrillation.

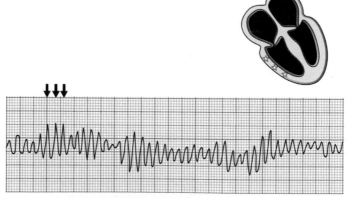

Fig. 21.2: Ventricular fibrillation: Irregular, bizarre and chaotic deflections

Clinical Relevance of Fast Irregular Bizarre QRS Rhythm

Ventricular Flutter

Ventricular flutter is very similar to ventricular tachycardia in terms of mechanism and causation. In fact, even their ECG features closely resemble each other and at times they are indistinguishable.

Nevertheless, conversion of ventricular tachycardia to ventricular flutter is often associated with a precipitous fall in cardiac output and blood pressure.

Most often, ventricular flutter is a very transient arrhythmia as it frequently and rapidly degenerates into ventricular fibrillation. Therefore, ventricular flutter is most often picked up during cardiac monitoring in intensive care units.

Since ventricular flutter almost always converts to ventricular fibrillation, it is the treatment of the latter condition that is required.

Ventricular Fibrillation

Ventricular fibrillation is the most feared of all arrhythmias. It is often a terminal catastrophic event with an exceedingly poor prognosis and invariable progression to death if untreated. It is also the most common cause of sudden cardiac death.

Primary ventricular fibrillation occurs in a patient who does not have pre-existing hypotension or heart failure while secondary ventricular fibrillation occurs in those who have these abnormalities. Underlying advanced myocardial disease is invariable in those who develop secondary ventricular fibrillation.

Local cellular and metabolic factors that predispose to ventricular fibrillation are hypoxia, acidosis, hypoglycemia, hyperkalemia, catecholamine excess and accumulation of free fatty acids or lactates.

Frequent causes of ventricular fibrillation are:
- Myocardial infarction
  - ➡ Acute
  - ➡ Old.
- Severe cardiomyopathy
  - ➡ Idiopathic
  - ➡ Ischemic.
- Drug intoxication
  - ➡ Digitalis
  - ➡ Quinidine.
- Metabolic derangement
  - ➡ Hypoxia
  - ➡ Acidosis.
- Accidental event
  - ➡ Electrical shock
  - ➡ Hypothermia.

Arrhythmias that are potentially serious as they may degenerate into ventricular fibrillation are:
- Ventricular tachycardia at more than 180 beats/minute
- Ventricular tachycardia with supervening ischemia
- Torsade de pointes due to prolonged QT interval
- VPCs demonstrating 'R-on-T' phenomenon
- Atrial fibrillation with an accessory pathway.

Differentiation between ventricular flutter and ventricular fibrillation is generally a futile exercise as flutter is transient and almost always degenerates into ventricular fibrillation.

Clinically, it may be difficult to differentiate between ventricular fibrillation and cardiac standstill or asystole as both conditions cause absence of peripheral pulses and heart sounds with loss of consciousness.

Nevertheless, their distinction is crucial, since defibrillation is required for ventricular fibrillation while external pacing is the mainstay of treatment for cardiac asystole.

The prognosis of ventricular fibrillation is exceedingly poor with invariable progress to death unless promptly treated. Prompt recognition and institution of defibrillation within a minute is the cornerstone of successful resuscitation.

Therefore, the prognosis of ventricular fibrillation is better for witnessed cardiac arrest in an intensive care unit or an operation theater with cardiac monitoring facility, than in the community.

Many victims of acute myocardial infarction can be rescued by training paramedical personnel and even laymen in the technique of cardiopulmonary resuscitation (CPR).

Moreover, mortality from myocardial infarction has declined in recent years through availability of intensive coronary care units (ICCUs) including mobile CCUs. These units are equipped with facilities for prompt recognition and cardioversion of serious ventricular arrhythmias, such as ventricular fibrillation.

The moment ventricular fibrillation is recognized, the immediate goal should be to restore an effective cardiac rhythm. If defibrillation equipment is not available, a vigorous blow may be given to the precordium. This is popularly known as 'thump version' and may occasionally succeed in restoring sinus rhythm.

If not, CPR should be begun immediately. Cardiac massage is done at a rate of 100 compresses per minute. After every 30 compresses, 2 artificial breaths are delivered to complete 5 such cycles in 2 minutes. The patient should be shifted to a hospital with intensive care and defibrillation facility, in the minimum possible time.

The likelihood of success of defibrillation declines rapidly with time and irreversible brain damage occurs within four minutes of circulatory collapse.

Electrical defibrillation with 200–360 Joules of DC shock is the procedure of choice for the treatment of ventricular fibrillation. Longer the duration of fibrillation, higher is the energy level of shock required.

If one attempt fails, defibrillation may be repeated after intravenous bicarbonate 1 mEq/kg to correct the underlying acidosis, which increases the success rate of cardioversion.

If repeated attempts at defibrillation fail, intravenous drugs should be given 30–60 second after each attempt. The dose of antiarrhythmic drugs that can be given is amiodarone 300 mg or lidocaine 1.0–1.5 mg/kg.

Recurrence of ventricular fibrillation can be prevented by antiarrhythmic drugs used for prevention of ventricular tachycardia. Drugs that are used include flecainide, phenytoin, propafenone and sotalol.

Implantable defibrillators are now available, which when given to an ambulatory patient, can automatically sense ventricular fibrillation and deliver an electrical shock. The device is known as Automatic Implantable Cardioverter Defibrillator or AICD.

Slow Regular Rhythm with Narrow QRS

REGULAR SLOW RHYTHM

A regular cardiac rhythm that occurs at a rate of less than 60 beats per minute indicates two broad possibilities:

- Slow discharge of impulses from the pacemaker governing the rhythm of the heart
- Block of alternate beats so that the conducted beats appear to occur at a slow rate.

If the discharge rate of impulses is slow, the focus of impulse origin is:

- Sinoatrial (SA) node
- Junctional pacemaker.

If alternate beats are blocked, the block is:

- Sinoatrial (SA) block
- Atrioventricular (AV) block
- Blocked atrial ectopic beats.

Narrow QRS complexes during such a rhythm indicate normal intraventricular conduction of impulses from a supraventricular pacemaker.

Let us examine the specific arrhythmias that are associated with these features.

SINUS BRADYCARDIA

The occurrence of sinus node discharge at a rate of less than 60 beats/minute constitutes sinus bradycardia **(Fig. 22.1)**.

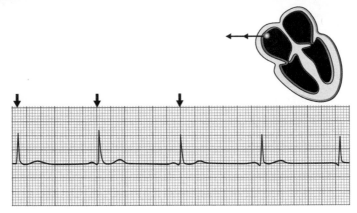

Fig. 22.1: Sinus bradycardia: Heart rate less than 60/min (RR >25 mm)

In other words, the RR interval exceeds 25 mm (heart rate = 1500/>25 = < 60). The rhythm is regular and the P wave and QRS morphology as well as P-QRS relationship are obviously as in normal sinus rhythm.

In case of hypothermia, there is wavering of the isoelectric line due to muscle twitching with shivering **(Fig. 22.2)**. The small hump at the end of the QRS complex or the beginning of the ST segment, is known as the J wave or the Osborne wave. Another cause of the J wave or Osborne wave is the early repolarization variant.

JUNCTIONAL ESCAPE RHYTHM

Junctional rhythm originates from a latent subsidiary pacemaker located in the AV junction. Normally, this pacemaker is subdued, when the cardiac rhythm is governed by the SA node. However, if the SA node is at fault (sinus pause or sinus arrest), this junctional pacemaker takes charge of the cardiac rhythm.

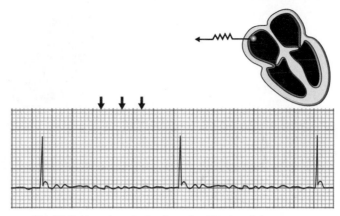

Fig. 22.2: Hypothermia: Bradycardia, shivering, Osborne wave

Junctional rhythm is an example of escape rhythm since the junctional pacemaker escapes the subduing influence of the SA node on the expression of its automaticity.

A junctional rhythm occurs at a rate of 40–60 beats/minute which is the inherent rate of the junctional pacemaker **(Fig. 22.3)**.

The distinctive feature of a junctional rhythm is the typical relationship between P waves and QRS complexes. As the atria are activated retrogradely, the P waves are inverted. They may just precede, just follow or be buried in the QRS complexes because of nearly simultaneous atrial and ventricular activation.

These characteristics of a junctional rhythm help to differentiate it from sinus bradycardia where the P waves are upright and always precede the QRS complexes by a fixed PR interval.

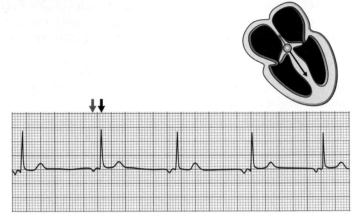

Fig. 22.3: Junctional rhythm: Inverted P-waves precede the QRS complexes

SINUS RHYTHM WITH 2:1 SA BLOCK

In second-degree sinoatrial block (2° SA block), there is inter-mittent dropping of beats, resulting in pauses. In a dropped beat, the entire P-QRS-T complex is missing as neither atrial nor ventricular activation occurs.

If the pattern of dropped beats is such that an alternate beat is missing (2:1 SA block), the conducted beats resemble a slow regular rhythm, such as sinus bradycardia.

The only difference is that if atropine is administered in 2:1 SA block, there is a sudden doubling of the heart rate while in sinus bradycardia the heart rate accelerates gradually.

SINUS RHYTHM WITH 2:1 AV BLOCK

In second-degree atrioventricular block (2° AV block), there is intermittent dropping of ventricular complexes, resulting in pauses. In a dropped beat, the P-wave is not followed by a QRS complex as atrial activation is not followed by ventricular activation.

If the pattern of dropped beats is such that an alternate QRS complex is missing (2:1 AV block), the normally conducted beats resemble a slow regular rhythm, such as sinus bradycardia or 2:1 SA block.

A 2:1 AV block can be differentiated from 2:1 SA block by the fact that P waves are recorded normally and only the QRS complexes are missing in alternate beats.

BLOCKED ATRIAL ECTOPICS IN BIGEMINY

An atrial premature complex (APC) inscribes a premature P-wave followed by a normal QRS complex and then a compensatory pause before the next sinus beat is recorded.

A very premature APC may find the AV node still refractory to ventricular conduction and may consequently get blocked. Such an APC inscribes a P-wave that deforms the T-wave of the preceding beat, is not followed by a QRS complex but followed by a compensatory pause.

If such blocked APCs alternate with normal beats, the normal sinus beats resemble a slow regular rhythm, such as sinus bradycardia or 2:1 SA block.

The distinctive feature of blocked atrial ectopics in bigeminal rhythm is the occurrence of premature bizarre P-waves deforming the T-waves.

A 2:1 AV block also produces blocked P-waves but they are not premature and are normal in morphology.

Clinical Relevance of Slow Regular Narrow QRS Rhythm

Sinus Bradycardia

Sinus bradycardia represents response of the SA node to a variety of physiological and pathological stimuli mediated by the nervous and hormonal control over the rate of pacemaker discharge.

The causes of sinus bradycardia are:

- Advanced age and athletic built
- Deep sleep and hypothermia
- Intracranial tension and glaucoma
- Hypopituitarism and hypothyroidism
- Obstructive jaundice and uremia
- Beta-blockers and verapamil
- Sick sinus syndrome
- Vasovagal syncope.

Sinus bradycardia is usually observed in young healthy persons, conditioned athletes and marathon runners who have parasympathetic dominance. It is also seen in elderly patients with sinus node dysfunction.

Sinus bradycardia during strenuous activity and in the absence of medical conditions or drugs likely to cause a slow heart rate is a sign of sinus-node dysfunction, the so called "sick sinus syndrome".

Sinus bradycardia is not a primary arrhythmia and therefore, treatment should be directed towards the basic underlying condition. Examples are hormone replacement in endocrinal disorders, decongestive therapy in high intracranial/intraocular tension, medical treatment of hepatic/renal disease and withdrawal of the offending drug in drug-induced sinus bradycardia.

Symptomatic sinus bradycardia in the absence of these conditions should be managed as sick sinus syndrome. Atropine and sympathomimetic drugs can temporarily accelerate the ventricular rate.

Junctional Rhythm

A junctional escape rhythm is a 'rescue' rhythm in which the junctional pacemaker is asked to govern the rhythm of the heart when the sinus node produces insufficient impulses due to severe bradycardia or SA block.

The term 'escape' rhythm signifies that the junctional pacemaker has escaped the subduing influence of the dominant pacemaker, the SA node. A junctional bradycardia after sinus arrest is the body's defence mechanism against prolonged asystole.

The causes of junctional bradycardia are:

- Normal in athletes
- Sinus node dysfunction
- Drug therapy
  - ⇒ Digoxin
  - ⇒ Amiodarone
  - ⇒ Diltiazem
  - ⇒ Beta-blockers.

Sinus Rhythm with 2:1 Block

A sinus rhythm in which alternate beats are blocked (2:1 block) closely resembles sinus bradycardia as the conducted beats appear to occur at a slow rate. The block may be either sinoatrial (SA block) or atrioventricular (AV block).

Sick sinus syndrome is a frequent cause of 2:1 SA block next only to drugs that reduce the pacemaker discharge rate (e.g. propranolol, diltiazem).

The causes of 2:1 AV block are acute carditis, drugs that cause 2:1 SA block (see above) and inferior wall myocardial infarction.

In the management of symptomatic 2:1 block, drugs like atropine and adrenaline can temporarily accelerate the ventricular rate.

Temporary cardiac pacing is effective in tiding over the crisis in acute carditis, drug toxicity or myocardial infarction.

Permanent cardiac pacing is the answer to the management of sick sinus syndrome when symptoms are severe, recurrent and long-standing.

Blocked APCs in Bigeminal Rhythm

Atrial premature complexes that are blocked in the AV node and alternate with sinus beats, resemble a slow rhythm. This occurs because of the compensatory pause that follows each premature beat.

Such a rhythm needs to be differentiated from other slow rhythms, the management of which is entirely different.

Blocked or nonconducted atrial premature beats are frequently observed in elderly patients who have advanced AV nodal disease and in the presence of digitalis toxicity.

Slow Irregular Rhythm
with Narrow QRS

IRREGULAR SLOW RHYTHM

An irregular cardiac rhythm that occurs at a rate of less than
60 beats per minute indicates three possibilities:
- Slow and variable rate of pacemaker discharge
- Beat-to-beat variability of the focus of origin
- Varying degree of conduction block of regular beats.

Narrow QRS complexes during such a rhythm indicate
normal intraventricular conduction of impulses from a
supraventricular pacemaker.

Let us examine the specific arrhythmias that are associated
with these features.

SINUS ARRHYTHMIA

Sinus arrhythmia is an irregular rhythm characterized by
periods of slow and fast heart rate due to variation in the rate
of SA node discharge.

When the periodic change in sinus rate is related to
the phases of respiration, it is known as respiratory sinus
arrhythmia. Nonrespiratory sinus arrhythmia is where the
sinus rate variability is uninfluenced by the respiratory cycle.

Sinus arrhythmia is characterized by alternating periods of
long and short PP and RR intervals reflecting a variable heart
rate **(Fig. 23.1)**.

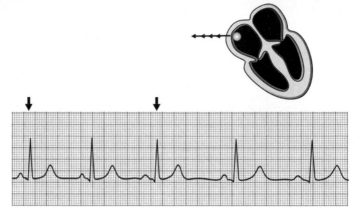

Fig. 23.1: Sinus arrhythmia: Heart rate varies with respiration

In respiratory sinus arrhythmia, about four complexes occur at one rate while the next four complexes occur at a different rate. The figure of 4 presumes that the respiratory rate is one-fourth of the heart rate. The rate is faster in inspiration and slower in expiration.

In nonrespiratory sinus arrhythmia, the variability of heart rate is nonphasic and unrelated to respiration.

Since, all beats arise from the SA node, the P-wave shape, QRS complex morphology and PR interval are constant. Sinus arrhythmia is frequently associated with sinus bradycardia.

WANDERING PACEMAKER RHYTHM

Wandering pacemaker is a rhythm wherein, impulses take origin from different foci besides the SA node. The pacemaker, so to say, wanders from one focus to the other, from beat-to-beat. The focus of origin may be the SA node, the atrial myocardium or the AV junction.

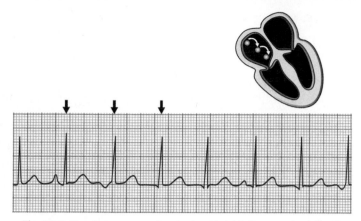

Fig. 23.2: Wandering pacemaker rhythm: Variable P-wave; changing PR interval

Wandering pacemaker rhythm is characterized by a beat-to-beat variability of the P-wave morphology **(Fig. 23.2)**.

Upright P-waves arise from the SA node or upper atrium while inverted P waves arise from the lower atrium or AV junction.

The PR interval also varies from beat-to-beat due to variability of the AV conduction time. Lower atrial or junctional beats have a shorter P-R interval because of shorter conduction time.

Multifocal atrial tachycardia (MAT) is also characterized by variability of P-wave morphology but the heart rate is 100–150 beats per minute. In wandering pacemaker rhythm, the heart rate ranges from 60–100 beats/minute.

Wandering pacemaker rhythm can be differentiated from sinus arrhythmia by the fact that the variability of heart rate is not phasic but on a beat-to-beat basis. Moreover, in sinus arrhythmia, the P-wave morphology and PR interval are constant, since all beats arise from the SA node.

SINUS RHYTHM WITH VARYING SA BLOCK

In second-degree sinoatrial block (2° SA block), there is intermittent dropping of beats, resulting in pauses. In a dropped beat, the entire P-QRS-T complex is missing as neither atrial nor ventricular activation occurs.

The pattern of dropped beats determines the conduction ratio, such as 2:1 SA block if alternate beats are dropped, 3:2 if every third beat is dropped and so on. If the conduction ratio is variable, it produces a slow irregular rhythm.

SINUS RHYTHM WITH VARYING AV BLOCK

In second-degree atrioventricular block (2° AV block), there is intermittent dropping of ventricular complexes, resulting in pauses. In a dropped beat, the P-wave is not followed by a QRS complex as atrial activation is not followed by ventricular activation.

The ratio of the number of P waves to number of QRS complexes determines the conduction sequence, such as 2:1 AV block if alternate P-wave is blocked, 3:2 if every third P-wave is blocked and so on. If the conduction ratio is variable, it produces a slow irregular rhythm.

Varying AV block can be differentiated from varying SA block by the fact that P waves are recorded normally in AV block. They are altogether missing along with the QRS complexes, in case of SA block.

Clinical Relevance of Slow Irregular Narrow QRS Rhythm

Sinus Arrhythmia

Respiratory sinus arrhythmia is produced by variation in the vagal tone in relation to the respiratory cycle, caused by reflex mechanisms in the pulmonary and systemic vasculature. It is a normal physiological phenomenon often observed in children and young athletic individuals.

Nonrespiratory sinus arrhythmia is an irregularity of heart rate produced by a dysfunctional SA node in elderly patients, the so called sick sinus syndrome.

Since sinus arrhythmia results from variation in the vagal influence on the SA node, it is accentuated by vago-tonic procedures like carotid sinus massage and abolished by vagolytic procedures, such as exercise and atropine administration.

Absence of sinus arrhythmia with a clock-like regularity of the heart rate indicates absence of vagal influence on the SA node and is a feature of cardiac autonomic neuropathy.

Lack of heart rate variability with a resting tachycardia is a feature of sympathetic dominance and carries high mortality in diabetic autonomic neuropathy.

It is also absent in atrial septal defect because of equalized left and right atrial pressures, with no effect of respiration on the vagal tone.

Respiratory sinus arrhythmia in children and young adults merits no active treatment. Nonrespiratory sinus arrhythmia in the elderly is managed as sick sinus syndrome.

Wandering Pacemaker Rhythm

A cardiac rhythm due to a wandering pacemaker is a striking but benign electrocardiographic abnormality. It is often observed in young, asymptomatic and healthy individuals.

Occasionally, wandering pacemaker rhythm is observed during the course of digitalis treatment or acute rheumatic fever.

No active treatment is indicated in young asymptomatic persons in whom a wandering pacemaker rhythm is observed incidentally.

Management of digitalis toxicity or rheumatic carditis is indicated if these causes are implicated. Symptomatic bradycardia due to this rhythm is managed with atropine or sympathomimetics.

Sinus Rhythm with Varying Block

A sinus rhythm, when complicated by sinoatrial or atrioventricular block of a variable degree, produces an irregular heart rate.

Sick sinus syndrome is a frequent cause of varying SA block. Variable AV block is often due to rheumatic carditis or acute inferior wall infarction.

Slow Atrial Fibrillation

Atrial fibrillation generally produces a fast irregular ventricular rhythm. This is because, out of the large number of fibrillatory waves, only a few can randomly penetrate the AV node and activate the ventricles producing a ventricular rate of 100–150 beats per minute.

In other words, atrial fibrillation is associated with a variable degree of physiological AV block. If this physiological

AV block is advanced, the ventricular rate is slow, resulting in slow atrial fibrillation.

Slow atrial fibrillation is observed, if there is preexisting AV nodal disease or during treatment with drugs like propranolol, verapamil or diltiazem that block the AV node.

Atropine and sympathomimetic agents can temporarily accelerate the ventricular rate in symptomatic SA or AV block.

Temporary pacing is useful in the acute phase of carditis, drug intoxication or myocardial infarction. Permanent cardiac pacing is the answer to recurrent and severe symptoms due to sick sinus syndrome.

Slow Regular Rhythm with Wide QRS

SLOW WIDE QRS RHYTHM

A regular cardiac rhythm that occurs at a rate of less than 60 beats per minute indicates slow discharge of impulses from the pacemaker governing the rhythm of the heart.

If the QRS complexes during such a rhythm are wide, two possibilities have to be considered:

- The rhythm is ventricular in origin in which case ventricular activation is through myocardium and not the specialized conduction system
- The rhythm is supraventricular in origin but there is a preexisting abnormality causing wide QRS complexes.

A slow ventricular rhythm occurs in these situations:

- Complete AV block with an idioventricular rhythm
- Complete SA block with ventricular escape rhythm
- Ventricular rhythm from an external pacemaker.

Let us go into the classical features of these rhythms.

COMPLETE AV BLOCK

In complete or third-degree atrioventricular block (3° AV block), there is a total interruption of AV conduction with the result that no sinus beat is able to activate the ventricles.

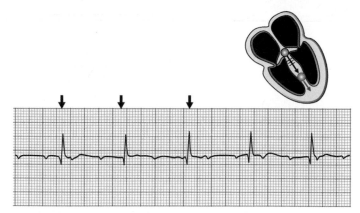

Fig. 24.1: Third-degree (complete) AV block: Wide QRS complexes

Therefore, the ventricles are governed by a subsidiary pacemaker in the ventricular myocardium. The inherent rate of this pacemaker is 20–40 beats per minute and hence, the wide QRS complexes occur at this rate **(Fig. 24.1)**.

However, since the atria continue to be activated by the SA node, the P waves occur at a rate of 70–80 beats per minute. Since, the SA node and the ventricular pacemaker are asynchronous and produce independent rhythms, there is no relationship between the P waves and QRS complexes. This is known as AV dissociation.

The ventricular rhythm at its inherent rate of 20–40 beats per minute is called idioventricular rhythm.

Occasionally in complete AV block, the ventricles are governed by a subsidiary pacemaker in the His bundle. The inherent rate of this pacemaker is 40–60 beats per minute and hence, the QRS complexes occur at this rate.

Moreover, since ventricular conduction proceeds through normal pathway, the QRS complexes are narrow **(Fig. 24.2)**.

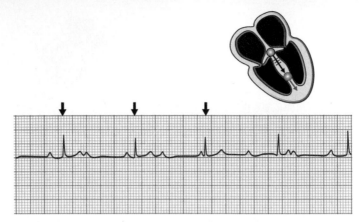

Fig. 24.2: Third-degree (complete) AV block: Narrow QRS complexes

A His bundle rhythm closely resembles a junctional rhythm as both occur at the same rate and produce narrow QRS complexes.

The differentiating feature is that in His bundle rhythm of complete AV block, the QRS complexes are unrelated to the P waves. In a junctional rhythm, the P waves just precede, just follow or are merged with the QRS complexes.

COMPLETE SA BLOCK

In complete or third-degree sinoatrial block (3° SA block), there is sinus node arrest or total atrial standstill with the result that ventricular activation is not possible.

Therefore, a subsidiary pacemaker comes to rescue by taking over the rhythm of the heart. Generally, it is the junctional pacemaker which governs the cardiac rhythm in this situation, known as junctional escape **(Fig. 24.3)**.

However, if the AV node is diseased, a ventricular pacemaker is called upon to govern the heart, producing a ventricular rhythm. The inherent rate of this pacemaker is

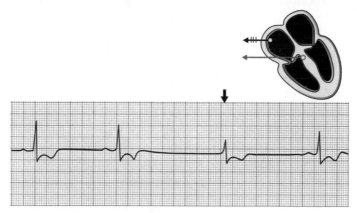

Fig. 24.3: Sinoatrial block followed by junctional escape

20–40 beats per minute and wide QRS complexes occur at this rate.

Since the ventricular pacemaker escapes the subduing influence of the SA node on the expression of its automaticity, the rhythm is known as ventricular escape rhythm.

A ventricular escape rhythm in complete SA block resembles the idioventricular rhythm in complete AV block as both occur at a similar rate and produce wide QRS complexes. They can be differentiated by the fact that normal P-waves at a rate of 70–80 beats continue to occur in AV block. No signs of atrial activation are observed in SA block and therefore, P-waves are altogether absent.

EXTERNAL PACEMAKER RHYTHM

In complete SA block or AV block with a very slow heart rate, the definitive form of treatment is implanting an external pacemaker. Artificial pacing is generally done from the right ventricle. The pacemaker is programmed to deliver impulses at a predetermined rate of around 60 beats per minute.

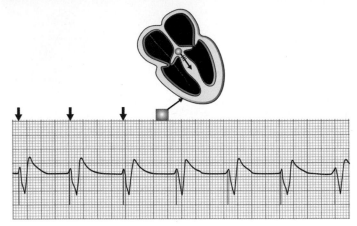

Fig. 24.4: External pacemaker rhythm: Spike before each QRS

These impulses are generated either continuously (fixed mode pacing) or intermittently (demand mode pacing) that is, only when the pacemaker senses an insufficient number of intrinsic impulses.

In either case, the pacemaker beats produce wide QRS complexes as the ventricles are activated asynchronously, right ventricular activation preceding the left. The heart rate depends upon the rate to which the pacemaker has been programmed.

The rhythm from an external pacemaker resembles an idioventricular rhythm of complete AV block. The differentiating feature is a spike-like deflection before each "captured" cardiac response, known as pacemaker artefact **(Fig. 24.4)**.

SLOW RHYTHM WITH PRE-EXISTING WIDE QRS COMPLEXES

It is known that certain conditions produce an abnormality of ventricular conduction even in sinus rhythm causing an alteration of QRS morphology.

Three well known examples are:

- Bundle branch block (complete)
- WPW syndrome (pre-excitation)
- Intraventricular conduction defect.

If a slow supraventricular rhythm, such as sinus bradycardia occurs in the presence of a preexisting QRS abnormality, it is naturally associated with wide QRS complexes.

A bundle branch block produces a triphasic QRS contour while an intraventricular conduction defect results in a bizarre QRS morphology. The WPW syndrome is characterized by a delta wave on the ascending limb of the QRS complex.

Clinical Relevance of Slow Regular Wide QRS Rhythm

Complete AV Block

The causes of complete or third-degree AV block are:

- Congenital heart disease, e.g. septal defect
- Coronary disease, e.g. anteroseptal infarction
- Cardiac surgery, e.g. atrial septal repair
- Aortic valve disease, e.g. calcific stenosis
- Fibrocalcerous degeneration, e.g. Lev's disease.

In complete AV block, the ventricles are governed by a subsidiary pacemaker in the His bundle or the ventricular myocardium. While a His bundle rhythm produces narrow QRS complexes at 40–60 beats/minute, a ventricular rhythm produces wide QRS complexes at 20–40 beats/minute.

A His bundle rhythm is more stable, reliable to sustain ventricular function, can be accelerated by atropine and rarely causes symptoms. On the other hand, a ventricular rhythm is unstable, unreliable to sustain ventricular function, cannot be accelerated by atropine and often causes syncope. Clinical importance of AV block depends upon:

- Causes of the AV block—reversible or irreversible
- Site of the lower pacemaker—His bundle or ventricle
- Symptomatology of the patient—present or absent.

The most common symptom of complete AV block is spells of dizziness or fainting due to transient ventricular asystole with sudden decline in cardiac output. Such episodes or syncopal attacks are known as Stokes-Adams attacks.

Other causes of Stokes-Adams attacks are:

- Complete sinoatrial block
- Serious ventricular arrhythmia
- Carotid sinus hypersensitivity
- Subclavian steal syndrome.

It is extremely important to differentiate Stokes-Adams attack due to complete AV block from that due to a ventricular arrhythmia as their management is entirely different. While asystole requires atropine or cardiac pacing, ventricular arrhythmia requires antiarrhythmic drugs or electrical cardioversion.

Complete AV block produces the following clinical signs that help to differentiate it from other slow rhythms:

- Dissociation of jugular venous waves from carotid arterial pulsations, due to AV dissociation
- Variable intensity of the first heart sound, due to variable duration of diastolic filling period.

Cardiac pacing is the definitive form of treatment in complete AV block. While temporary pacing may be enough to tide over a transient situation, such as an acute myocardial infarction or a postoperative complication, permanent pacing is the answer to a chronic condition like calcific degeneration of the AV node.

Pacing is invariably required in these situations:

- Wide QRS rhythm at less than 40 beats/minute
- History of recurrent Stokes-Adams attacks
- Setting of an acute myocardial infarction.

Complete SA Block

The causes of complete or third-degree SA block are:
- Drug therapy, e.g. propranolol, digitalis, diltiazem
- Vagal stimulation, e.g. by carotid sinus pressure
- Sinus node dysfunction, e.g. sick sinus syndrome.

In complete SA block, the ventricles are governed by a subsidiary pacemaker in the AV junction or the ventricular myocardium. While a junctional rhythm produces narrow QRS complexes at 40–60 beats/minute, a ventricular rhythm produces wide QRS complexes at 20–40 beats/minute.

Both these rhythms are examples of an escape rhythm, since the subsidiary pacemaker escapes the subduing influence of the SA node on the expression of its automaticity. A ventricular escape rhythm occurs only if the AV node is diseased and cannot govern the cardiac rhythm.

Sinoatrial block may coexist with atrioventricular block and even right or left bundle branch block especially in elderly individuals with a diffuse fibrocalcerous or degenerative process involving the entire conduction system.

The escape rhythm in complete SA block is a "rescue" rhythm in the absence of which prolonged asystole would invariably result in death.

The most common symptom of complete SA block is spells of dizziness or fainting due to transient ventricular asystole along with sudden decline in cardiac output. SA block in one of the causes of Stokes-Adams attacks.

Treatment of symptomatic individuals involves administration of drugs like atropine and sympathomimetic drugs to accelerate the heart rate. The dosages of these drugs used are:

Atropine 0.6 mg IV; repeat every 3–5 minute up to response or a total dose of 0.03–0.04 mg/kg

OR

Isoprenaline infusion at 1–4 μg/minute

Cardiac pacing remains the definitive form of treatment of complete SA block. When the SA block is a part of sick sinus syndrome, the management of that condition is indicated.

External Pacemaker Rhythm

The artificial pacemaker is an electronic device that can generate impulses to activate the heart, if the intrinsic rhythm is slow or unstable. Generally, the pacemaker lead with the electrode as its tip is implanted on the endocardial surface of the right ventricle.

External pacing may be employed temporarily to tide over an acute transient situation or permanently in a chronic condition.

There are two modes of cardiac pacing namely, fixed-mode pacing and demand-mode pacing.

In fixed-mode pacing, impulses are generated at a predetermined rate, irrespective of the intrinsic rhythm. In demand-mode pacing, the pacemaker generates impulses intermittently on demand, when it senses a slow intrinsic rhythm.

When an external pacemaker governs the cardiac rhythm, the ventricles are not activated synchronously but sequentially. The right ventricle is activated before the left since the pacing electrode is located in the right ventricle.

Therefore, an artificial pacemaker rhythm is characterized by wide QRS complexes. The rate of the pacemaker rhythm is the rate at which the pacemaker has been programmed.

Slow Rhythm with Existing Wide QRS

The occurrence of a slow rhythm in a patient who has a preexisting condition causing wide QRS complexes, such as bundle branch block or conduction defect, understandably simulates an idioventricular rhythm.

The availability of a previous ECG during normal sinus rhythm that reveals wide QRS complexes can settle the issue.

Moreover, the triphasic contour of a bundle branch block or the delta wave of WPW syndrome are too characteristic to be mistaken for the wide QRS complexes of a ventricular rhythm.

Interesting Cases Diagnosed by ECG

CASE 1:
LEFT VENTRICULAR HYPERTROPHY

A 56-year-old obese gentleman visited his physician with the complaints of frequent headaches and spells of dizziness. He also found it difficult to carry out routine tasks and felt fatigued and breathless even on mild physical exertion. The patient was diagnosed to have systemic hypertension about 30 years back. At that time, he was extensively investigated for secondary hypertension, but no renal or endocrine disorder was detected. He was prescribed antihypertensive medications, but did not take them regularly and was not on periodic medical follow-up.

On examination, the patient was grossly overweight, with a body mass index (BMI) of 34 kg/m². The pulse was regular, good in volume and the heart rate was 84 beats/minute. All peripheral pulses were palpable and there was no carotid bruit or brachiofemoral delay. The BP was 164/106 mm Hg over the right arm in the sitting position. The S1 was normal but the A2 sound was accentuated; a S4 sound was heard in presystole. An ECG was obtained (**Fig. 25.1**).

The ECG showed tall R waves exceeding 25 mm in the left precordial leads and deep S waves in the right precordial leads. There also was ST segment depression and T-wave

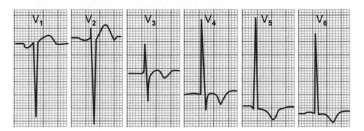

Fig. 25.1: ECG showing tall R waves in left chest leads with deep S waves in right chest leads

inversion in the lateral leads. These findings are consistent with the diagnosis of left ventricular hypertrophy. The tall R waves in the lateral precordial leads, reflect the increased electrical forces generated by the thickened left ventricular myocardium. S-T segment depression and T wave inversion in these leads indicate left ventricular strain. Additional findings can include notched bifid P waves (P. mitrale) due to left atrial enlargement and left axis deviation of the QRS vector.

Voltage criteria are often employed for the electrical diagnosis of left ventricular hypertrophy **(Table 25.1)**. The Sokolow and Lyon criteria of S in V1 plus R in V5 or V6 greater than 35 mm is popularly used. Another criteria used is of Framingham wherein, R in V5 or V6 >25 mm or R in aVL >11 mm is taken as criteria for left ventricular hypertrophy. The left ventricular (LV) strain pattern of ST segment depression and T-wave inversion is observed in LV pressure overload. In

TABLE 25.1: Voltage criteria for left ventricular hypertrophy

· **Sokolow and Lyon criteria** S. in V_1 + R in V_5 or V_6 >35 mm
· **Framingham criteria** R in V_5 or V_6 >25 mm; R in aVL >11 mm

TABLE 25.2: Causes of left ventricular hypertrophy

Systolic overload
• Aortic valve stenosis
• Systemic hypertension
• Coarctation of the aorta
• Hypertrophic cardiomyopathy
Diastolic overload
• Mitral regurgitation
• Aortic incompetence
• Ventricular septal defect
• Patent ductus arteriosus

case of LV volume overload, the S-T segment is isoelectric and the T wave is upright and tall.

Causes of left ventricular hypertrophy are classified into those of systolic overload and the causes of diastolic overload. Systolic overload is due to systemic hypertension, aortic stenosis, coarctation of aorta and hypertrophic cardiomyopathy. Causes of diastolic overload are mitral and aortic valve regurgitation and an intracardiac left-to-right shunt, such as ventricular septal defect or patent ductus arteriosus **(Table 25.2)**.

Left ventricular hypertrophy is an independent predictor of cardiovascular morbidity and mortality, as a risk factor for myocardial infarction, stroke, heart failure and sudden arrhythmic death. Serial echoes are performed annually to monitor the progress of hypertensive heart disease, particularly to assess the regression of LVH with antihypertensive drug therapy.

Current practice guidelines recommend that all hypertensive patients with left ventricular hypertrophy, target organ damage and associated cardiovascular risk factors particularly diabetes, should be offered antihypertensive drug treatment. The choice of first-line therapy has been the subject of debate, as well as the study design of several clinical trials. It is being believed that newer agents like calcium channel blockers (e.g. amlodipine) or an ACE inhibitor (e.g. ramipril) are more effective for regression of hypertrophy than older agents like diuretics (e.g. thiazide) or beta-blockers (e.g. atenolol).

CASE 2:
LEFT BUNDLE BRANCH BLOCK

A 63-year-old man was brought to the emergency room past midnight, with the complaint of shortness of breath and difficulty in lying flat on the bed. The patient had sustained an anterior wall myocardial infarction 5 months back and ever since, he had complained of easy fatiguability and dyspnea on exertion. For the past 1 week, he required 2 or 3 pillows in bed to catch sleep and yet woke up often because of air-hunger.

On examination, the patient was obviously tachypneic and looked anxious. He was pale and diaphoretic. The extremities were cold but there was no cyanosis. The pulse was fast and low in volume. The BP was 104/74 mm Hg over the right arm in the supine position. The cardiac apex beat was diffuse and displaced towards the left axilla. The S_1 was normal and the A_2 was loud. There was paradoxical splitting of S_2. A S_3 was also appreciated in early diastole. Auscultation over the lung fields revealed bilateral crepts over the bases posteriorly. An ECG was obtained **(Fig. 25.2)**.

The ECG showed broad ventricular complexes, that measured 0.14 second in width. In leads L_1 and V_6, each ventricular complex had two peaks, producing a M-shaped RsR' pattern. The broad complex was followed by ST segment depression and T-wave inversion. These findings are consistent with the diagnosis of left bundle branch block. Bundle branch block denotes delayed or interrupted conduction down the right or left branch of the bundle of His **(Fig. 25.3)**. It leads to widening of the ventricular complex, due to delayed

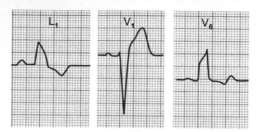

Fig. 25.2: ECG showing wide QRS complexes due to left bundle branch block

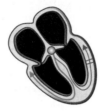

Fig. 25.3: Diagram to represent left bundle branch block (LBBB)

depolarization of the ventricle whose bundle branch is blocked. The QRS complexes of both the ventricles are "out of sync" with each other and produce two R waves in sequential order. Incomplete bundle branch block (BBB) results in QRS width of 0.11 to 0.12 second while in complete BBB, the QRS width exceeds 0.12 second. The ST segment depression and T-wave inversion are repolarization abnormalities, secondary to the abnormal pattern of ventricular depolarization.

In left bundle branch block (LBBB), the M-shaped RsR' pattern is observed in lead V6. The notched R wave represents abnormal sequence of septal and left ventricular free wall depolarization. There is total distortion of the normal QRS complex. In right bundle branch block (RBBB), the M-shaped rsR pattern is observed in lead V1. The septal (denoted by r) and free wall (denoted by S) depolarization through the left bundle branch are normal. Right ventricular depolarization

TABLE 25.3: Causes of left bundle branch block

- Myocardial infarction
- Aortic valve stenosis
- Systemic hypertension
- Dilated cardiomyopathy
- Fibrocalcerous degeneration

(denoted by R') is delayed. Therefore, RBBB does not distort the normal QRS complex, but only adds a terminal R' deflection.

Left bundle branch block (LBBB) often indicates the presence of organic heart disease. A variety of cardiac conditions can cause LBBB including myocardial infarction, systemic hypertension, aortic valve disease, cardiomyopathy and fibrocalcerous degeneration **(Table 25.3)**. On the other hand, right bundle branch block (RBBB) is sometimes observed in normal individuals. Typical causes of RBBB are atrial septal defect, acute pulmonary embolism and chronic obstructive pulmonary disease.

Right bundle branch block (RBBB) does not distort the QRS complex, but only adds a terminal deflection due to delayed right ventricular depolarization. Therefore, changes of myocardial infarction, such as appearance of Q waves and loss of R wave height, can be readily diagnosed in the presence of RBBB. However, it is difficult to diagnose myocardial infarction in the presence of LBBB, since the QRS complex is completely distorted. The criteria for the diagnosis of myocardial infarction in the presence of LBBB is given in **Table 25.4**.

There is no specific treatment of left bundle branch block. The underlying heart disease is to be managed on its own merit. There is a word of caution regarding the use of drugs which block the AV node, such as verapamil, diltiazem

TABLE 25.4: Criteria for diagnosing MI in presence of LBBB

- Presence of q wave in L_1, V_5 and V_6
- Terminal S wave in leads V_5 and V_6
- ST segment drift greater than 5 mm
- Upright T wave concordant with QRS

and beta-blockers. They may cause complete heart block, particularly if the block is bifasicular or trifasicular to begin with. Bifasicular block includes right bundle branch block and left anterior hemiblock. Trifasicular block is bifasicular block with a prolonged PR interval.

CASE 3:
FEATURES OF HYPOKALEMIA

A 48-year-old man sought consultation from a physician for pain and weakness in both arms, since the last 3 days. There was no history of chest pain, breathlessness, palpitation or sweating. The heaviness in the arms was aggravated by lifting a light weight, but not by movement at the neck. The patient also complained of fatigue and pain over his calf muscles while walking. He had systemic hypertension for several years for which he was presently prescribed losartan 50 mg and hydrochlorthiazide 25 mg. The patient also suffered from bronchial asthma, for which he used an inhaler containing a combination of salmeterol and fluticasone. Recently, he had a gastrointestinal infection with profuse vomiting and diarrhea that lasted 2 days. Besides age and hypertension, other cardiovascular risk factors in the patient were prediabetes and a modestly elevated serum cholesterol. An ECG was obtained **(Fig. 25.4)** following which he was asked to immediately see a cardiologist. His blood biochemistry was glucose 128 mg/

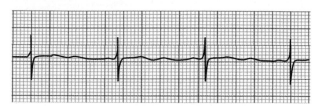

Fig. 25.4: ECG showing flat T waves with prominent U waves

dL, urea 38 mg/dL, creatinine 1.2 mg/dL, LDL cholesterol 147 mg/dL, sodium 131 m Eq/L and potassium 2.9 mEq/L.

The ECG showed normal sinus rhythm. The P wave and QRS complex were normal in morphology. There were no significant Q waves and the ST segment was isoelectric. The T wave was reduced in amplitude, while the U wave was prominent. The QT interval seemed to be prolonged. These findings are consistent with the diagnosis of hypokalemia. Hypokalemia is an important cause of T wave change. The T wave is either reduced in amplitude, flattened or inverted. This is associated with prominence of the U wave that follows the T wave. The low T wave followed by a prominent U wave produces a 'camel-hump' effect.

In hypokalemia, the T wave is flattened and the prominent U wave may be mistaken for the T wave. This may falsely suggest prolongation of the QT interval, whereas it is actually the QU interval. Hypokalemia, therefore, causes pseudo-prolongation of the QT interval, at the expense of T wave. The U wave that is exaggerated and approximates the size of the T wave is considered to be a prominent U wave. Other causes of prominent U wave are cardiovascular drugs e.g. digitalis, quinidine and psychotropic agents, e.g. phenothiazines, tricyclic antidepressants.

The ECG features of hypokalemia depend upon its severity (**Fig. 25.5**). In mild hypokalemia, only the T wave amplitude is reduced. In moderate hypokalemia, the U wave becomes more prominent than the T wave. In severe hypokalemia,

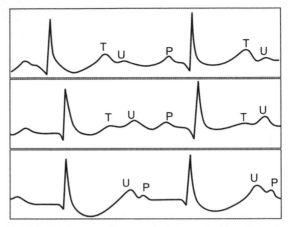

Fig. 25.5: ECG features of progressively increasing hypokalemia

TABLE 25.5: ECG features of progressive hypokalemia

• Reduced amplitude of the T wave
• Flat T wave with prominent U wave
• ST segment sagging; only U wave

there is sagging of the ST segment and only the U wave is visible **(Table 25.5)**.

There are several causes of hypokalemia which have been enlisted in **Table 25.6**. True loss of potassium is due to vomiting, diarrhea, nasogastric suction and diuretic therapy. Redistribution of potassium occurs in metabolic alkalosis (intracellular shift) and with beta-agonist or insulin therapy. Hypokalemia is a feature of cortisol excess due to Cushing's disease or steroid therapy as well as a feature of hyperaldosteronism in Conn's syndrome. Genetic causes of hypokalemia are Type 2 renal tubular acidosis (RTA-2) and hypokalemia periodic paralysis. Typical clinical features of hypokalemia are fatigue and leg cramps. In severe cases,

TABLE 25.6: Causes of hypokalemia

Body fluid loss
- Diuresis
- Vomiting
- Diarrhea

Redistribution
- Metabolic alkalosis

Drug-induced
- Beta-agonist
- Insulin therapy

Hyperaldosteronism
- Cushing's disease
- Conn's syndrome

Genetic causes
- Hypokalemic periodic paralysis
- Renal tubular acidosis Type 2

neuromuscular paralysis and cardiac arrhythmias may occur. In cardiac patients on diuretic treatment, hypokalemia aggravates digitalis toxicity and increases the likelihood of serious ventricular arrhythmias.

In our case, the hypokalemia was multifactorial. Firstly, the patient was prescribed a diuretic for his hypertension. Secondly, he was using an inhaled beta-agonist for asthma, which is known to cause hypokalemia. Finally, he had a recent bout of gastroenteritis, which might have caused substantial loss of potassium from his body.

Management of hypokalemia includes potassium replacement and correction of the underlying cause. Potassium can be replaced through dietary supplementation of potassium-rich foods. Oral proprietary supplements of potassium citrate can also be prescribed. If potassium deficiency is severe or if the patient is vomiting, potassium chloride is administered as an intravenous infusion. Generally, potassium deficiency is more severe, if there is true loss of body fluids than if there is only a transcellular shift of potassium.

CASE 4:
FEATURES OF HYPERKALEMIA

A 64-year-old woman was wheeled into the emergency room, with generalized weakness and shortness of breath of one week duration. She also complained of swelling around the eyes and over the feet, loss of appetite and occasional vomiting. The lady was a known case of diabetes mellitus since 25 years and systemic hypertension for the last 12 years. She sustained an anterior wall myocardial infarction four years back, for which she was thrombolysed. At that time, coronary angiography showed triple-vessel disease, but she declined a revascularization procedure. Her serum creatinine value was found to be high and therefore, she was switched over from oral antidiabetic drugs to insulin therapy. The patient also underwent laser photocoagulation for proliferative retinopathy, one year back. She was presently undergoing maintenance hemodialysis, thrice a week.

An ECG was obtained **(Fig. 25.6)** following which she was immediately given an injection. Her laboratory reports were hemoglobin 9.2 g/dL%, urine sugar +1 albumin +2, glucose 144 mg/dL, urea 124 mg/dL, creatinine 5.2 mg/dL, sodium 129 mEq/L, potassium 6.8 mEq/L and calcium 7.4 mg%.

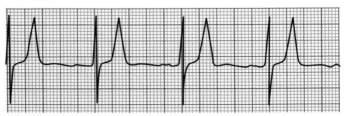

Fig. 25.6: ECG showing tall T waves with flat P waves

The ECG showed normal sinus rhythm. The P wave was flattened and the PR interval was prolonged. There were no significant Q waves and the ST segment was isoelectric. The T wave was upright, tall and peaked. The QT interval was short. These findings are consistent with the diagnosis of hyperkalemia. A T-wave that exceeds a voltage of 5 mm in the standard leads and 10 mm in the precordial leads is considered tall. Besides hyperkalemia, causes of tall T wave are myocardial ischemia and the hyperacute phase of myocardial infarction. The T wave of hyperkalemia is tall, peaked symmetrical and has a narrow base, the so called 'tented' T wave. The QT interval is short. On the other hand, the T wave of coronary insufficiency is tall but broad-based and the QT interval is prolonged.

The normal QT interval is 0.39 + 0.04 second and ranges from 0.35 to 0.43 second. A QT interval measuring less than 0.35 second is considered short. Besides hyperkalemia, causes of short QT interval are hypercalcemia and digitalis toxicity. Hyperkalemia shortens the QT interval and is associated with tall T waves, wide QRS complexes and diminished P waves. Hypercalcemia also shortens the QT interval but there are no changes in the morphology of the QRS deflection. The proximal limb of the T-wave has an abrupt upslope to its peak.

The ECG features of hyperkalemia depend upon its severity **(Fig. 25.7)**. When the serum level exceeds 6.8 mEq/L, tall T waves and short QT interval are seen. When it exceeds 8.4

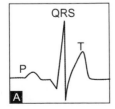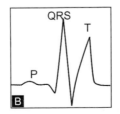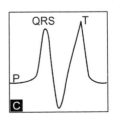

Fig. 25.7: ECG features of progressively increasing hyperkalemia

mEq/L, additionally the P wave gets flattened and the P-R interval gets prolonged. At a serum level which is in excess of 9.1 mEq/L, the QRS complex also becomes wide and ventricular arrhythmias occur **(Table 25.7)**.

There are several causes of hyperkalemia which have been enlisted in **Table 25.8**. True gain of potassium is often due to hemolysis, rhabdomyolysis, burns or tumor lysis. Redistribution of potassium occurs in metabolic

TABLE 25.7: ECG features of progressive hyperkalemia

A.	Serum K >6.8 mEq/L	Tall T waves; Short QT interval
B.	Serum K >8.4 mEq/L	(A) plus flat P waves; Prolonged PR interval
C.	Serum K >9.1 mEq/L	(B) plus wide QRS complex; AV block and arrhythmias

TABLE 25.8: Causes of hyperkalemia

Potassium gain
- Hemolysis, tumor lysis
- Rhabdomyolysis, burns

Redistribution
- Metabolic acidosis
- Hyperglycemia

Hypoaldosteronism
- Addison's disease
- Acute renal failure

Drug-induced
- Potassium sparing diuretics
- Nonsteroidal anti-inflammatory drugs
- Antiangiotensin drugs (ACEi & ARBs)

Genetic causes
- Hyperkalemic periodic paralysis
- Renal tubular acidosis Type 4

acidosis (extracellular shift), with beta-blocker therapy and in severe insulin deficiency. Hyperkalemia is a feature of hypoaldosteronism due to Addison's disease or acute on chronic renal failure. Drugs known to cause hyperkalemia include potassium-sparing diuretics, nonsteroidal anti-inflammatory drugs (NSAIDs), and the angiotensin converting enzyme (ACE) inhibitors. Genetic causes of hyperkalemia are Type 4 renal tubular acidosis (RTA-4) and hyperkalemic periodic paralysis.

The clinical picture of hyperkalemia depends upon the cause. The most common scenario is of acute on chronic renal failure with fluid overload, hypertension and metabolic acidosis, which are characteristic features of uremia. Sometimes, hyperkalemia is a part of diabetic ketoacidosis. At other times, burns and crush-injuries with rhabdomyolysis are associated with hyperkalemia. Severe hyperkalemia can cause serious ventricular arrhythmias.

Since hyperkalemia can cause serious ventricular arrhythmias, the first priority is to protect the heart. Calcium gluconate has membrane stabilizing properties and is administered intravenously as 10 mL of 10% injection over 10 minutes. The next step is to drive potassium into the cells using 100 mL of 25% glucose with 10 units of insulin given by an infusion. Nebulized salbutamol increases the urinary excretion of potassium by increasing the Na-K-ATPase pump activity. Excess potassium in the body can be depleted by potassium-binding resin like polystyrene sulphonate administered orally. Finally, if severe hyperkalemia is associated with metabolic acidosis and fluid overload, hemodialysis is the answer.

CASE 5:
PROLONGED QT SYNDROME

A 62-year-old woman visited her cardiologist along with her daughter, because of two episodes of syncope in the preceding week. The fainting episodes were preceded by palpitation and associated with blurring of vision. The patient was a known case of coronary heart disease and she had sustained an anterior wall myocardial infarction 10 months back. The patient also felt breathless on exertion and her echocardiogram showed a large anterior wall motion abnormality with an ejection fraction of 30 ± 5%. About a month back, she underwent 24-hour Holter monitoring which showed multifocal ventricular premature beats, with short runs of ventricular tachycardia. Therefore, she was prescribed amiodarone, in addition to her usual medication which included ramipril, frusemide, aspirin, atorvastatin and isosorbide mononitrate. An ECG was obtained **(Fig. 25.8).**

The ECG showed normal regular sinus rhythm. The P waves were normal in morphology and large Q waves were seen in the anterior precordial leads. The T wave was upright, tall and broad, which occupied most of the RR interval. The measured QT interval was 0.60 second. This finding is consistent with the diagnosis of long QT syndrome.

The duration of the QRS complex represents ventricular depolarization time and the width of the T wave represents

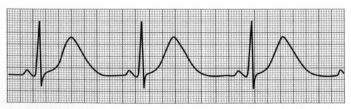

Fig. 25.8: ECG showing broad T waves with prolonged QT interval

ventricular repolarization time. Therefore, the QT interval is a measure of the total duration of ventricular electrical systole. The QT interval is measured on the horizontal axis, from the onset of the Q wave to the termination of the T wave (not the U wave). The duration of the QRS complex, the length of the ST segment and the width of the T wave are included in the measurement of the QT interval.

The upper limit of normal QT interval depends upon several variables, including the age, gender and the autonomic tone. It tends to be shorter in young individuals (0.44 sec) and longer in the elderly (0.45 sec). It is slightly shorter in males than in females, the upper limit being 0.43 second in men. The QT interval shortens at fast heart rates and lengthens at slow heart rates. Since the QT interval varies with tachycardia and bradycardia, the measured QT interval needs to be corrected for heart rate.

The corrected QT interval is known as the QTc interval. For heart rate correction, the Bazett's formula is generally used, where QTc interval is equal to the measured QT interval divided by the square-root of the RR interval. When the heart rate is 60 beats/minute and the RR interval is 1 second (25 × 0.04 second), the QTc interval and the QT interval are the same. As a general rule, a QT interval that exceeds half of the R-R interval, is taken as a prolonged QT interval.

There are several causes of QT interval prolongation. These have been enlisted in **Table 25.9**. Congenital long QT syndromes may present dramatically with syncope. Indeed, congenital long QT syndromes are characterized by prolongation of the QT interval, syncope, 'seizures' and sudden death due to ventricular arrhythmias (Torsade de pointes), in apparently healthy children and young adults. Some cases of sudden infant deaths have been attributed to congenital long QT syndrome. Therefore, an ECG should be performed in all infants on anticonvulsants for seizure

TABLE 25.9: Causes of prolonged QT interval

Congenital causes
- Jervell-Lange-Neilsen syndrome
  (autosomal recessive with deafness)
- Romano-Ward syndrome
  (autosomal dominant without deafness)

Acquired causes
- Electrolyte deficiency, e.g. calcium, potassium
- Antiarrhythmic drugs, e.g. quinidine, amiodarone
- Coronary artery disease, e.g. myocardial infarction
- Myocarditis, e.g. viral myocarditis, rheumatic fever
- Intracranial event, e.g. head injury, brain hemorrhage
- Bradyarrhythmias, e.g. AV block, sinus bradycardia
- Drug-induced, e.g. terfenadine, cisapride, olanzapine

prophylaxis. The prognosis and triggers of sudden cardiac death in patients with congenital long QT syndrome, are related to the QT interval and the genotype.

Antiarrhythmic drugs, such as quinidine, procainamide and amiodarone can prolong the QT interval. They also cause widening of the QRS complex which, if it exceeds 25% of baseline, is an indication for withdrawing the culprit drug. Since QT interval prolongation predisposes to arrhythmias, this is the mechanism to explain the arrhythmia enhancing property or proarrhythmic effect of antiarrhythmic drugs. Besides antiarrhythmic agents, certain non-cardiovascular drugs can also prolong the QT interval. These drugs are listed in **Table 25.10**.

The clinical importance of QT interval prolongation lies in the fact that it predisposes to a typical type of polymorphic ventricular tachycardia. This tachycardia is known as "Torsade de pointes", a ballet term which literally means "torsion around a point". This term explains the morphology of the ventricular tachycardia, which consists of polymorphic QRS complexes

TABLE 25.10: Drugs causing QT interval prolongation

Antiarrhythmics	Anti-infectives
• Quinidine • Procainamide • Amiodarone	• Erythromycin • Gatifloxacin • Ketoconazole
Psychiatry drugs	**Miscellaneous drugs**
• Imipramine • Haloperidol • Amitryptyline	• Cisapride • Terfenadine • Ketanserin

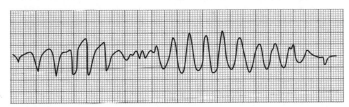

Fig. 25.9: Polymorphic ventricular tachycardia ('Torsade de pointes')

that keep changing in amplitude and direction **(Fig. 25.9)**. The polymorphic QRS complexes give the appearance of periodic torsion or twisting around the isoelectric line.

Long QT syndrome (LQTS) belongs to a class of congenital channelopathies, that are responsible for about 5–10% cases of sudden cardiac death (SCD). Other conditions belonging to this class are the Brugada syndrome and catecholaminergic ventricular tachycardia (CVT). Besides these above channelopathies, structural heart diseases responsible for SCD are hypertrophic cardiomyopathy and arrhythmogenic right ventricular dysplasia.

The treatment of long QT syndrome depends upon the cause. When the cause is reversible, it suffices to correct the electrolyte abnormality or to withdraw the offending drug. The QT interval should be carefully assessed at peak plasma concentration, if multiple drugs with QT prolonging effect are used. In QT interval prolongation due to a cardiovascular or intracranial event, the underlying condition has to be managed. Since patients with congenital long QT syndrome are prone to syncope and sudden death due to ventricular arrhythmias, an implantable cardioverter defibrillator (ICD) is advocated.

CASE 6:
SICK SINUS SYNDROME

A 78-year-old elderly gentleman was paid a domiciliary visit by his physician, to evaluate frequent spells of dizziness over the past 2 weeks. The patient felt light-headed when he stood up from the sitting or lying down position. Fortunately, he had never fallen down or fainted because he used a walking aid and was regularly looked after by a personal attendant. There was no history of breathlessness, chest pain or palpitation. The patient was hypertensive for over 40 years and took his medicines regularly. There was no past history of myocardial infarction or paralytic stroke. The only time he was hospitalized was for prostate surgery five years back. The patient's family members had also noticed recent mental confusion and lapses in his memory.

An ECG was obtained **(Fig. 25.10)**. At the time of prostate surgery, an ECHO had shown mild concentric left ventricular hypertrophy with an ejection fraction of 52% and no regional

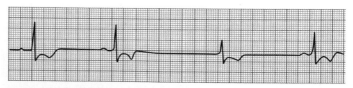

Fig. 25.10: ECG showing sinus bradycardia, asystole and junctional escape

wall motion abnormality. CT scan of the head at the same time showed periventricular lacunar infarcts and changes of diffuse cerebral atrophy.

The ECG showed sinus bradycardia at a rate of 50 beats/minute, with short periods of asystole. At times the RR interval was twice the usual RR interval, suggesting 2:1 sinoatrial exit block (SA block). At other times, the period of asystole was followed by a delayed beat without a preceding P wave, consistent with a junctional escape beat. This constellation of ECG findings which includes sinus bradycardia, SA block and junctional escape, is consistent with the diagnosis of sinus node dysfunction, the so called sick sinus syndrome **(Table 25.11)**.

The sick sinus syndrome usually presents with bradyarrhythmias, such as those mentioned above. At times the indications of sinus node dysfunction are an inadequate tachycardia with sympathomimetic drugs, excessive sensitivity to beta-blocker drugs and atropine resistant bradycardia. At other times, there may be atrial fibrillation with slow ventricular response or a junctional rhythm. The coexistence of fast and slow cardiac rhythms constitutes the classical "tachy-brady" syndrome.

Quite often, sinus node dysfunction is suspected clinically but difficult to prove because the ECG is normal and Holter monitoring does not show up the arrhythmia, during the period of observation. A prolonged sinus node recovery time (SNRT) and sinoatrial conduction time (SACT) on

TABLE 25.11: ECG findings in sick sinus syndrome

· Sinus bradycardia
· Sinoatrial exit block
· Slow atrial fibrillation
· Junctional escape rhythm

electrophysiological studies (EPS) is then taken as a diagnostic criteria for sick sinus syndrome (SSS).

The "sick sinus syndrome" (SSS) is a clinical condition caused by a diseased sinus node, which fails to produce or successfully conduct a sufficient number of cardiac impulses. It is observed in elderly patients and is believed to be caused by a degenerative condition like amyloidosis or infiltration of the atrium by a fibrocalcerous process. Certain cardiovascular drugs notably beta-blockers (atenolol, metoprolol), calcium-blockers (verapamil, diltiazem) and digoxin may also cause sinus node dysfunction, which is reversible after discontinuation of therapy.

The most frequent symptoms of sick sinus syndrome are dizziness, mental confusion and fainting attacks (Table 25.12). Spells of dizziness and syncope in sick sinus syndrome are due to transient ventricular asystole, causing a precipitous decline in stroke volume and cerebral perfusion. Such episodes are known as Stokes-Adams attacks. Besides SSS, other causes of Stokes-Adam's attacks are advanced atrioventricular block, malignant ventricular arrhythmias, carotid sinus hypersensitivity and subclavian steal syndrome (Table 25.13).

Since patients are in the advanced age group, many of them have had a cerebrovascular accident or a prior myocardial infarction. They may also complain of dyspnea and fatigue due to heart failure. Palpitation and angina pectoris may occur due to tachyarrhythmias or associated coronary artery disease. Dizziness and syncope in an elderly

TABLE 25.12: Symptoms of sick sinus syndrome

· Dizziness and syncope
· Dyspnea and fatigue
· Palpitation and angina
· Confusion and dementia

TABLE 25.13: Causes of Stokes-Adams attacks

- Advanced atrioventricular block
- Serious ventricular arrhythmias
- Carotid sinus hypersensitivity
- Subclavian steal syndrome
- Sick sinus syndrome

patient may be multifactorial. Even those with documented sick sinus syndrome may additionally have volume depletion, electrolyte imbalance or hypoglycemia. They may have orthostatic hypotension due to autonomic failure or vertebro-basilar insufficiency. Still others may have cardiac outflow obstruction due to aortic sclerosis or ventricular arrhythmias due to an old myocardial scar or heart failure. Therefore, a detailed evaluation of these patients is warranted.

Drugs that can increase the rate of discharge from the sinus node, such as sympathomimetic (adrenaline) and vagolytic (atropine) drugs, can only temporarily increase the heart rate. Permanent pacemaker implantation (PPI) is the definitive form of treatment, particularly if the symptoms are severe and disabling. Dual-chamber pacemakers are more physiological and carry a lower risk of atrial fibrillation and stroke. They also have a distinct advantage over single-chamber pacing if there is coexistent AV nodal disease or bundle branch block. Pacemaker implantation makes it possible to use antiarrhythmic drugs to treat tachyarrhythmias, which otherwise would have caused severe bradycardia.

CASE 7:
EARLY REPOLARIZATION SYNDROME

A 29-year-old well-built man of African origin, sought an appointment with the cardiologist, for opinion on an abnormal ECG. The ECG was performed as a part of routine pre-employment medical evaluation. The man vehemently denied complaints of fatigue, breathlessness, chest pain, palpitation or syncope. He had been actively involved in competitive sports during his college days and still played tennis on week-ends. The man did not smoke or take alcohol, but was fond of calorie-dense food. He did not suffer from diabetes or hypertension and had never got a serum lipid analysis done.

On examination, the man was of stocky built, with a muscular physique. His body mass index (BMI) was 28 kg/m^2. The pulse rate was 58–62 beats/minute. with a normal pulse volume and no special character. The BP was 120/80 mm Hg over the right arm. The precordium was unremarkable, with a normally located apex beat. The S_1 and S_2 were normal without any gallop sound. No murmur or pericardial friction rub was audible. A fresh ECG was performed in the cardiologist's office **(Fig. 25.11)**.

The ECG showed tall R waves in the lateral precordial leads, preceded by narrow Q waves. The ST segment was elevated concave upwards, with an initial slur on the ST segment (J wave). The T waves were upright, tall and symmetrical in the lateral leads, with prominent U waves in the mid-precordial leads. These findings are consistent with the diagnosis of early repolarization syndrome **(Table 25.14)**. Since early

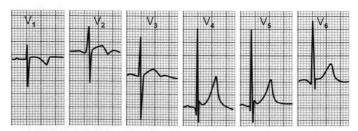

Fig. 25.11: ECG showing features of early repolarization syndrome

repolarization is frequently observed in healthy athletic persons, this entity is also known as the "athlete's heart".

There are several causes of ST segment elevation **(Table 25.15)**, of which acute myocardial infarction is the leading cause. The ST segment elevation of early repolarization, can simulate the injury pattern of acute myocardial infarction. However, there are several classical differentiating features:

- ST segment elevation is concave upwards in lead V_6
- Ratio of ST elevation: T wave height is below 0.25
- There is no reciprocal ST depression in other leads
- ECG changes do not evolve as in case of infarction
- ECHO does not show abnormal regional wall motion
- Serial level of cardiac enzyme titers does not increased.

TABLE 25.14: ECG features of early repolarization syndrome

Tall R wave in lead V_6
Narrow and deep Q wave
Concave ST segment elevation
Initial J wave on the ST segment
Upright and tall symmetrical T wave

TABLE 25.15: Causes of ST segment elevation

Coronary artery disease
Myocardial infarction
Prinzmetal's angina
Dressler's syndrome
Ventricular aneurysm
Noncoronary disease
Acute pericarditis
Pulmonary embolism
Early repolarization
Brugada syndrome

The "early repolarization" variant is an alarming electro-cardiographic entity, which presents with ST segment elevation. It represents early repolarization of a portion of the ventricle, before the entire myocardium has been depolarized. There is an early uptake of the ST segment, before the descending limb of the R wave has reached the baseline. This causes an initial slur on the ST segment, known as the J wave. The ST segment is elevated and concave upwards. There is an associated increased amplitude of the R wave. The T wave is also tall, but the ratio of ST segment elevation to T wave height is less than 0.25. Interestingly, the degree of ST elevation and T wave height may vary on a day-to-day basis and the ST segment may normalize after exercise. Besides the features already mentioned, other characteristics of this syndrome are sinus bradycardia with sinus arrhythmia, voltage criteria of left ventricular hypertrophy and persistent juvenile pattern of T wave inversion in leads V_1 to V_3.

Early repolarization is more frequently observed among young athletic males of Africo-Carribean descent. They are healthy subjects who are free of symptoms and their clinical examination is entirely normal. Acute viral pericarditis also presents with concave-upwards ST segment elevation but sinus tachycardia is almost invariably present. Moreover, patients of acute pericarditis have a preceding flu-like illness, they present with chest pain and there is an audible pericardial rub.

Individuals who have features of early reploarization on the ECG, are healthy asymptomatic subjects without any objective evidence of organic heart disease. Therefore, no specific treatment apart from reassurance is advocated. However, lack of awareness about this entity may lead to unnecessary investigations including stress-testing, myocardial perfusion imaging and coronary angiography.

CASE 8:
BRUGADA SYNDROME

A 28-year-old man was asked to see a cardiologist by a general physician, for expert opinion on an abnormal ECG. The ECG had been performed by the physician empanelled with an insurance company, as part of the pre-insurance medical check-up. The man clearly denied any history of chest pain, dyspnea, palpitation or syncope. He was physically very active and undertook a brisk walk for 40 minutes, on most days of the week. He had also been a regular member of his school and college cricket teams. The man smoked about 5 cigarettes a day and consumed about 1 liter of beer on week-ends. His blood pressure and blood sugar levels were normal but his lipid profile showed an elevated LDL value. One of his cousin brothers had died of cardiac arrest, at the age of 32 years. A fresh ECG was obtained in the office of the cardiologist (**Fig. 25.12**).

The ECG showed a triphasic rSR' pattern in lead V_1, which was 0.10 second in duration. Additionally, there was a "tent-like" coved ST segment elevation of 0.2 mV with large inverted T waves (**Table 25.16**). These findings are consistent with the diagnosis of Brugada syndrome. Three types of ST segment elevation are described in Brugada syndrome, depending upon the ventricular repolarization pattern.

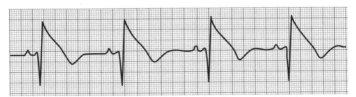

Fig. 25.12: ECG showing features of the Brugada syndrome

TABLE 25.16: ECG features of Brugada syndrome

• rSR' pattern in lead V_1
• rSR' duration <0.12 sec
• Large and inverted T wave
• Coved ST segment elevation

- **Type 1:** "Tent-like" coved ST segment, elevation >0.2 mV, negative T wave
- **Type 2:** "Saddle-back like" ST segment, elevation >0.1 mV, positive T wave
- **Type 3:** "Saddle-back like" ST segment, elevation <0.1 mV, positive T wave.

Besides Brugada syndrome, other causes of ST segment elevation in lead V_1 are right ventricular infarction, acute pulmonary embolism and arrhythmogenic right ventricular dysplasia **(Table 25.17)**. The rSR pattern in lead V_1 observed in case of Brugada syndrome, superficially resembles right branch block (RBBB). But unlike in RBBB, the ventricular complex is not more than 0.12 second wide and there are no broad S waves in lead L_1 and V_6. The characteristic ECG abnormalities observed in Brugada syndrome may only be transient and not observed constantly. These may become exaggerated or unmasked after drug challenge with antiarrhythmic agents, such as flecainide and procainamide.

TABLE 25.17 : Causes of ST segment elevation in lead V_1

• Brugada syndrome
• Right ventricular infarction
• Acute pulmonary embolism
• Arrhythmogenic RV dysplasia

The Brugada syndrome is a rare but striking electro-cardiographic abnormality. It is believed to be a genetic disorder of sodium transport, across ion channels located in the right ventricle. This produces an abnormal pattern of right ventricular depolarization. Patients who have this abnormality are prone to develop sudden syncope because of malignant ventricular tachycardia or even cardiac arrest due to ventricular fibrillation. The genetic defect underlying Brugada syndrome may exist in more than one family member and form the basis of familial ventricular arrhythmias. The disorder is transmitted down subsequent generations by autosomal dominant inheritance.

Brugada syndrome belongs to a class of congenital channelopathies which are responsible for nearly 5–10% cases of sudden cardiac death (SCD). Other members of this class are long QT syndrome (LQTS) and catecholaminergic ventricular tachycardia (CVT), as given in **Table 25.18.** Besides these channelopathies, congenital structural heart diseases responsible for SCD are hypertrophic cardiomyopathy and arrhythmogenic right ventricular dysplasia.

There is no specific treatment of the underlying disorder in Brugada syndrome. However, insertion of an automatic implantable cardioverter defibrillator (AICD) may be considered in those patients with history of recurrent syncope, after cardiac resuscitation from ventricular fibrillation, or if there is history of sudden cardiac death in a family member.

TABLE 25.18: Congenital channelopathies

• Brugada syndrome
• Long QT syndrome
• Catecholaminergic VT* (*ventricular tachycardia)

CASE 9:
WPW SYNDROME

A 24-year-old unmarried female arrived at the emergency-room, with the complaints of palpitation and light-headedness for the last 15 minutes. She drove herself to the hospital and admitted that she felt dizzy while driving. The patient also gave history of several such episodes in the past. At times, she was able to abort the attack by splashing cold water on her face, or by applying firm pressure over the eyes. At other times, she had to rush to the hospital, as on that day. The onset of these episodes was unrelated to physical exercise, emotional stress or to the intake of any particular food or beverage. There was no history of tremor, heat-intolerance, undue fatigue or significant weight-loss.

On examination, the patient was apprehensive but not tachypneic. The extremities were not cold but her palms were sweaty. The pulse rate was extremely rapid and exceeded 150 beats/minute, although it could not be counted accurately. The BP was 91/64 mm Hg over the right arm and she was apyrexial. There was no goitre, bruit over the thyroid gland or any clinical sign of Grave's disease. The attending doctor performed right carotid sinus massage which resulted in sudden termination of the patient's symptoms and a remarkable change in her heart rate. An ECG was obtained afterwards (Fig. 25.13).

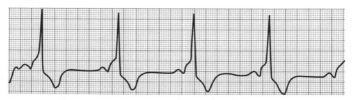

Fig. 25.13: ECG showing features of the WPW syndrome

The ECG showed normal P waves with a PR interval of 0.08 second. The width of the QRS complex was 0.12 second with a notch on the ascending limb of the R wave. There was depression of the ST segment with inversion of the T wave. These findings are consistent with the diagnosis of WPW syndrome. The Wolff-Parkinson-White (WPW) syndrome is a distinct electrocardiographic entity wherein an accessory pathway, the bundle of Kent, directly connects the atrial myocardium to the ventricular myocardium, bypassing the AV node **(Fig. 25.14).** This produces abnormalities of the QRS complex, PR interval, ST segment and the T wave.

The PR interval is short because ventricular depolarization through the accessory pathway, bypasses the normal conduction delay at the AV node. The notch on the ascending limb of R wave is the delta wave. It indicates preexcitation of the ventricle through the accessory pathway, before depolarization of the entire ventricle by the normal conduction system. The QRS complex is wide because it is a fusion beat, which is the sum of ventricular pre-excitation and normal ventricular depolarization. The ST segment and T wave inversion are repolarization abnormalities, secondary to the abnormal pattern of ventricular depolarization.

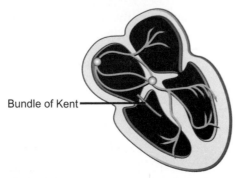

Bundle of Kent

Fig. 25.14: Diagram to illustrate the bundle of Kent

Three types of QRS configuration are described in the WPW syndrome, depending upon the direction of the accessory pathway.

- Type A (left septal connection) produces upright QRS complexes in all the precordial leads. It resembles right bundle branch block or true posterior wall myocardial infarction
- Type B (right-sided connection) has negative QRS complexes in V_1 and positive complexes in lead V_6. It resembles left bundle branch block or left ventricular hypertrophy
- Type C (left lateral connection) has positive QRS complexes in lead V_1 and negative complexes in lead V_6. It resembles right ventricular hypertrophy.

The WPW syndrome is a masquerader of several other cardiac conditions:

- The delta wave as separate from the R wave can mimic bundle branch block
- The dominant R wave in lead V_1 may resemble right ventricular hypertrophy
- Negative delta wave with ST segment depression and T wave inversion, may appear as myocardial infarction
- Antidromic AV re-entrant tachycardia conducted anterogradely through the accessory pathway may be mistaken for ventricular tachycardia.

Presence of the WPW syndrome predisposes an individual to paroxysmal supraventricular tachycardia (PSVT), wherein the bypass tract constitutes a re-entrant circuit along with the normal conduction pathway. In almost 90% patients, conduction proceeds anterogradely down the AV node and returns retrogradely through the accessory pathway to the atrium. This is known as orthodromic tachycardia and here the QRS complex is narrow. This arrhythmia responds to vagal maneuvers and to drugs used in the treatment of AV nodal reentrant tachycardia (AVNRT). These drugs include verapamil, diltiazem, digitalis and adenosine.

In less than 10% patients, anterograde conduction proceeds down the accessory pathway and returns retrogradely through the normal AV nodal pathway to the atrium. This is known as antidromic tachycardia and here the QRS complex is wide and demonstrates the WPW syndrome. This arrhythmia does not respond to vagal maneuvers, but only to cardioversion with DC shock or to antiarrhythmic drugs that block the accessory pathway, such as amiodarone.

CASE 10:
SUPRAVENTRICULAR TACHYCARDIA

A 36-year-old woman had been experiencing episodes of "fluttering" sensation in the chest, since 2 years. The episodes were described as a "machine-like" feeling over the precordium, that was not accompanied by chest pain or shortness of breath. During these episodes she did feel dizzy, but she never lost her consciousness. Once the episode was over, she would pass urine frequently. Her episodes were unrelated to physical exertion, food intake or to mental stress. At times she was able to abort the attack on her own, either by splashing cold water on her face or by applying firm pressure over her eyes. At other times, she had to visit a cardiologist who either performed carotid sinus massage or administered intravenous diltiazem. Initially, episodes would occur only once in a month or two but recently, their frequency had increased significantly. Therefore, although she was prescribed verapamil 120 mg twice a day which she took regularly, the patient was advised to undergo electrophysiological studies (EPS). A long-strip ECG recording of lead L_{II} was obtained (**Fig. 25.15**).

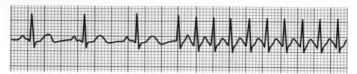

Fig. 25.15: ECG showing abrupt onset of narrow QRS tachycardia

The ECG showed an abrupt onset of regular tachycardia at a rate exceeding 150 beats/minute, with an RR interval of less than 10 mm. The QRS complexes were narrow and the P or T waves were not visible. These findings are consistent with the diagnosis of paroxysmal supraventricular tachycardia (PSVT).

Supraventricular tachycardia is most often (in 90% cases) based on repetitive circus movement of impulses in a closed reentrant circuit (reentrant tachycardia). In 50% cases, the circuit is composed of two pathways within the atrioventricular node [AV nodal reentrant tachycardia (AVNRT)]. In 40% cases, the circuit consists of an AV nodal pathway and an accessory bypass tract along its side [AV reentrant tachycardia (AVRT)]. An atrial impulse first passes anterogradely down one of the two pathways, the other pathway being in the refractory period. The impulses then returns retrogradely through the other pathway, which has by now recovered its conductivity. In this way, repetitive circulation of impulses occurs, to produce a sustained atrial tachycardia. Least often (in about 10% cases), supraventricular tachycardia is due to rapid discharge of impulses from an ectopic atrial focus (ectopic atrial tachycardia).

The heart rate in paroxysmal atrial tachycardia is 150–200 beats per minute, if a reentrant circuit is involved. It tends to be slower in ectopic atrial tachycardia (120–150 beats/minute), as the AV node cannot conduct more than 150 atrial impulses per minute. The heart rate can exceed a rate of

200 beats/minute, if an accessory bypass tract is involved, as in case of WPW syndrome. This is because in WPW syndrome, the impulses can bypass the decremental influence of the AV node, by traveling down the accessory pathway.

Most often, a supraventricular tachycardia is characterized by narrow QRS complexes, due to synchronized ventricular activation through the specialized His bundle conduction system. Occasionally, the supraventricular impulses find one of the two bundle branches refractory to conduction. In that case, the impulses are conducted only through the other bundle branch, producing a situation of aberrant ventricular conduction. This needs to be differentiated from a wide QRS ventricular tachycardia. The differences between ventricular tachycardia and supraventricular tachycardia with aberrant ventricular conduction are given in **Table 25.19.**

TABLE 25.19: Differences between ventricular tachycardia and supraventricular tachycardia with aberrant ventricular conduction

	Ventricular tachycardia	*SVT with aberrancy*
Regularity of rhythm	Slightly irregular	Clock-like
P waves	Not seen	May be seen
P-QRS relationship	Unrelated	Related
QRS width	>0.14 second	0.12–0.14 second
QRS morphology	Bizarre	Triphasic
QRS in V_1 to V_6	rS in V_1 to V_6	RsR' in V_1; Rs in V_6
RR' height	R > R'	R' > R
QRS axis	Leftward	Normal
Capture/fusion beats	May be seen	Not seen
Hemodynamics	Compromised	Stable
Organic heart disease	Often present	Often absent
Response to carotid massage	No response	Termination

Paroxysmal reentrant atrial tachycardia is most often based on a reciprocal mechanism involving a bypass tract or a dual intranodal pathway. Episodes of atrial tachycardia are one of the manifestations of preexcitation (WPW syndrome). In the absence of WPW syndrome, paroxysmal atrial tachycardia (PAT) is generally not associated with organic heart disease. If properly managed, PAT does not alter life-expectancy and carries an excellent prognosis. PAT coexisting with the WPW syndrome carries a poorer prognosis, because of the risk of degeneration into ventricular tachycardia. A paroxysm of atrial tachycardia in the presence of an underlying WPW syndrome is suggested, if it meets one of the following criteria:

- ECG during sinus rhythm shows short PR interval and wide QRS complex
- The ventricular rate exceeds 200 beats/minute, indicating the absence of a physiological AV block
- Inverted P waves are observed indicating retrograde atrial activation.

Symptoms due to atrial tachycardia depend upon the atrial rate, the duration of the tachycardia and the presence of heart disease. A fast atrial tachycardia causes palpitation and neck pulsations. Angina pectoris may occur due to increased myocardial oxygen demand and reduced coronary filling time. Prolonged atrial tachycardia can cause dizziness or syncope due to decline in cardiac output (shortened ventricular filling time) and loss of atrial contribution to ventricular filling. Termination of the tachycardia is often followed by polyuria due to the release of atrial natriuretic peptide (ANP) by the stretching of atrial myocardium.

The first step in the management of supraventricular tachycardia is to attempt vagal stimulation, to block the atrio-ventricular (AV) node. Vagal maneuvers include carotid sinus massage, supraorbital pressure, Valsalva maneuver and splashing ice-cold water on the face. If vagal maneuvers fail to abort the tachycardia, a drug to block the AV node is administered intravenously. Drugs that are effective include adenosine, diltiazem and amiodarone. After restoration of sinus rhythm, oral diltiazem, verapamil, amiodarone or a beta-blocker, such as metoprolol is prescribed to prevent recurrence.

The management of paroxysmal atrial tachycardia in the presence of WPW syndrome, is somewhat different. Vagal maneuvers are useful, only if anterograde conduction proceeds through the AV node. Digitalis is contraindicated as it enhances conduction down the accessory pathway and may precipitate ventricular fibrillation. Diltiazem and metoprolol reduce the tolerance to the high ventricular rate and can precipitate congestive heart failure. Amiodarone is the antiarrhythmic agent of choice for the long-term treatment and prevention of arrhythmias associated with the WPW syndrome.

The availability of sophisticated electrophysiological studies (EPS) to identify and locate bypass tracts and the development of latest ablative techniques, have revolutionized the management of WPW syndrome. For ablation of the bypass tract, high-frequency AC current is delivered through a thermister tipped catheter, which leads to localized heat coagulation. Radiofrequency ablation (RFA) of the bypass tract can be offered to patients who report recurrent and frequent symptomatic episodes of PAT which are refractory to drug therapy or those that cause hemodynamic compromise.

CASE 11:
ATRIAL FIBRILLATION

A 42-year-old woman presented with the complaints of palpitation and extreme fatigue. She denied history of chest pain or dizziness, but she felt tired and breathless after routine activities. During the preceding 6 months, she had unintentionally lost 4–5 kg of weight, despite having a good appetite. There was no history of excessive thirst or frequent urination, but she passed 3 to 4 semiformed stools everyday. The patient felt particularly uncomfortable during the summer months when her restlessness, fatigue and palpitations increased considerably.

On examination, the patient was restless, anxious and tachypneic. Her extremities were warm and her palms were dry. The pulse was fast, irregular and of good volume, with a pulse rate of 90–100 beats/minute. The heart rate by auscultation was 110–20 beats/minute, with a BP of 144/92 mm Hg over the right arm. Her temperature was 99.2ºF and the respiratory rate was 24/min. There was tremor over her outstretched hand and the eye-balls were prominent with lid retraction. The JVP was not raised and there were no palpable lymph nodes, but the thyroid gland was diffusely enlarged. The goiter was not tender, but a bruit was audible. A long-strip ECG recording of lead L_{II} was recorded (**Fig. 25.16**).

The ECG showed a fast irregular rhythm, with a variable RR interval. The QRS complexes were narrow, but no P waves were visible. Instead, there were fine fibrillatory waves between the QRS complexes. These findings are consistent with the diagnosis of atrial fibrillation (AF). Atrial fibrillation is a grossly irregular fast rhythm produced by functional fractionation of the atria into numerous tissue islets, in various stages of excitation and recovery. Consequently, atrial activation is chaotic and ineffectual in causing atrial

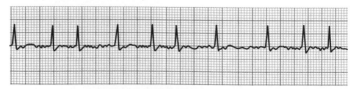

Fig. 25.16: ECG showing irregular rhythm with fine fibrillatory waves

contraction **(Fig. 25.17)**. Although 400 to 500 fibrillatory impulses reach the AV node per minute, only 100 to 150 of them succeed in eliciting a ventricular response, while others are blocked in the AV node. The random activation of the ventricles produces a grossly irregular ventricular rhythm.

The hallmark of atrial fibrillation is the absence of discrete P waves. Instead, there are numerous, small, irregular fibrillatory waves (f waves) that are difficult to identify individually but produce a ragged baseline. In long-standing atrial fibrillation, these undulations are minimal and produce a nearly flat baseline. As mentioned, the ventricular rate is grossly irregular and varies from 100 to 150 beats per minute. Atrial fibrillation can be differentiated from atrial flutter by the absence of P waves and an irregular ventricular rate **(Table 25.20)**. At times, precise differentiation between the two may be difficult and the rhythm is then known as "flutter-fibrillation", "coarse fibrillation" or "impure flutter".

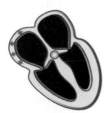

Fig. 25.17: Diagram to illustrate chaotic atrial activation

TABLE 25.20: Differences between atrial flutter and atrial fibrillation

	Atrial flutter	*Atrial fibrillation*
Atrial rate	220–350 beats/minute	Over 350 beats/minute
Ventricular rate	Regular. Half to one fourth of atrial rate	Variable. No relation to atrial rate
Atrial activity	Flutter (F) waves Saw-toothed baseline	Fibrillatory (f) waves Ragged baseline
Ventricular activity	Constant RR interval	Variable RR interval

In atrial fibrillation, the ventricular rate generally varies from 100 to 150 beats per minute. Faster rates are observed in children, patients of thyrotoxicosis and in the presence of WPW syndrome. Slower rates are observed during drug treatment with beta-blockers (propranolol, atenolol) or calcium-blockers (verapamil, diltiazem), as these drugs block the AV node. Elderly patients with AV nodal disease may also manifest slow atrial fibrillation. Regularization of the ventricular rate in a patient on digitalis for atrial fibrillation, indicates the onset of junctional tachycardia and is a manifestation of digitalis toxicity.

Atrial fibrillation (AF) can be classified into three groups. In paroxysmal AF, discrete episodes are self-terminating and last less than 48 hours. In persistent AF, fibrillation continues unabated for at least 7 days, but can be converted to sinus rhythm by electrical or chemical cardioversion. In permanent AF, fibrillation continues indefinitely and conversion to sinus rhythm is not possible. Atrial fibrillation can occur in virtually any form of heart disease. Common causes of AF are given in **Table 25.21**.

TABLE 25.21: Causes of atrial fibrillation

Persistent atrial fibrillation
- Dilated cardiomyopathy
- Constrictive pericarditis
- Cardiac trauma/surgery
- Hypertensive heart disease
- Valvular heart disease (MS)
- Coronary artery disease (MI)
- Congenital heart disease (ASD)

Paroxysmal atrial fibrillation
- Thyrotoxicosis
- WPW syndrome
- Sick sinus syndrome
- Lone atrial fibrillation
- Acute alcoholic intoxication
- Pulmonary thromboembolism

The symptoms of AF depend upon the ventricular rate, the nature and severity of underlying heart disease and the effectiveness of treatment. Palpitation is due to fast heart rate while syncope is caused by reduced cerebral perfusion. Angina may occur because of increased myocardial oxygen demand as well as shortened coronary filling time due to tachycardia. Dyspnea is due to pulmonary congestion, secondary to loss of atrial contribution to ventricular filling. Sometimes, regional ischemia in the form of limb gangrene, hemiparesis or blindness may occur because of systemic embolization from a left atrial thrombus.

Atrial fibrillation can be recognized clinically by several subtle signs. The pulse is irregularly irregular, with the pulse rate on palpation being less than the heart rate on auscultation (pulse deficit). The 'a' waves are not observed in the neck veins. There is a beat-to-beat variability in the pulse pressure as well as the intensity of first heart sound, because of a variable ventricular diastolic filling period.

The treatment of atrial fibrillation (AF) is governed by the patient's symptoms and hemodynamic status. In the majority of patients, long-term rate control along with oral anticoagulation, is a reasonable therapeutic strategy. Drugs that prolong the refractory period of the atrioventricular (AV) node, such as digoxin, diltiazem and metoprolol are effective for rate control in persistent AF. In patients of paroxysmal AF with infrequent episodes, a "pill in the pocket" (taken when symptomatic) strategy is preferable. Drugs used for this purpose are amiodarone, sotalol, flecainide and propafenone.

Long-standing atrial fibrillation produces stasis of blood in the left atrium and promotes the development of thrombi in the atrial cavity and the atrial appendage. Dislodged fragments of these thrombi can enter the systemic circulation as emboli and settle down in any arterial territory. Anticoagulants, such as caumarin and warfarin are required for long-term use in chronic atrial fibrillation, to reduce the likelihood of systemic embolization. This particularly applies to patients with rheumatic heart disease and to prosthetic valve recipients. Those patients with a previous history of thromboembolism (stroke or TIA) and those who have a documented atrial thrombus, are also candidates for long-term anticoagulant therapy.

If the patient's clinical status is poor and hemodynamics are unstable, electrical cardioversion with 100–200 Joules of energy is the treatment of choice, in an attempt to restore sinus rhythm. There are two requisites before cardioversion is attempted. Firstly, the patient should not have received digitalis in the previous 48 hours. Digitalis not only decreases the threshold for defibrillation, but also predisposes to the risk of life-threatening arrhythmias. Secondly, an oral anticoagulant should be initiated before cardioversion and continued for at least 4 weeks. This is because atrial thrombi are more likely to dislodge as emboli, once sinus rhythm is restored. Cardioversion should not be attempted if there is a documented left atrial clot.

In patients who are symptomatic but either refractory or intolerant to several antiarrhythmic agents, the final option is of radiofrequency ablation (RFA). Advantages of RFA are not only freedom from symptoms but also avoidance of the toxic effects of antiarrhythmic drugs and the need to monitor anticoagulant therapy.

CASE 12:
VENTRICULAR TACHYCARDIA

A 66-year-old woman was brought to the emergency department with history of recurrent syncope preceded by palpitation and dizziness. She had sustained an anterior wall myocardial infarction 8 months back and also complained of exertional breathlessness with paroxysms of nocturnal dyspnea. She did not receive thrombolytic therapy and had not undergone primary angioplasty because she presented to the hospital, over 24 hours after the onset of chest pain. The patient was practically home-bound with limited physical activity and did not complain of exertional angina. An echocardiogram was performed a month after her myocardial infarction, which revealed a large wall motion abnormality involving the mid and distal septum, ventricular apex and the distal lateral wall. The left ventricular ejection fraction was 25%. Along with a 12-lead ECG, a rhythm strip of lead LII was obtained, which showed an alarming but transient abnormality (Fig. 25.18).

The ECG rhythm strip showed an abrupt onset of irregular tachycardia, at a rate of about 200 beats/minute, with RR interval of 7–8 mm. The QRS complexes were bizarre and wide, exceeding 0.14 sec in width, but did not conform to a bundle branch block pattern. The P and T waves were not discernable. These findings are consistent with the diagnosis of ventricular tachycardia. Ventricular tachycardia is due to enhanced automaticity of a latent ventricular pacemaker, that fires impulses rapidly. Alternatively, it is based on a closed reentrant circuit around a fixed anatomical substrate in the ventricular myocardium (Fig. 25.19). Ventricular tachycardia may be sustained (lasting >30 sec) or nonsustained (lasting <30 sec). It is classified as monomorphic (similar QRS

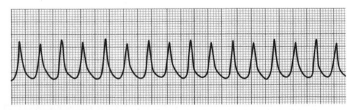

Fig. 25.18: ECG strip showing monomorphic ventricular tachycardia

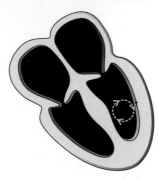

Fig. 25.19: Diagram to illustrate ventricular reentrant circuit

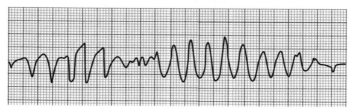

Fig. 25.20: ECG showing polymorphic ventricular tachycardia

complexes) or polymorphic (variable QRS complexes) in nature.

Polymorphic ventricular tachycardia is characterized by phasic variation of the QRS direction. A series of ventricular complexes are first up-pointing then down-pointing and this phenomenon occurs in a repetitive continuum **(Fig. 25.20)**. Since this gives the appearance of rotation around the isoelectric line, it is called "Torsade de pointes", a ballet term which literally means "twisting around a point". Torsade de pointes is generally, associated with prolongation of the QT interval. The prolonged QT interval favors the occurrence of a ventricular premature beat that coincides with the T-wave of the preceding beat (R-on-T phenomenon) and initiates the ventricular tachycardia.

How to Report an ECG

HOW TO REPORT AN ECG

Having gone through the various potential abnormalities in the ECG graph, it would be worthwhile to understand how a routine ECG is formally reported.

The first thing to note in the graph is the heart rate. The heart rate is determined from the RR interval. A short RR interval indicates tachycardia, while a long interval denotes bradycardia.

Normally, the rhythm of the heart originates from the sinoatrial (SA) node and is known as a sinus rhythm. Alternatively, the rhythm may arise from the atrial myocardium (atrial rhythm) or from the atrioventricular (AV) node called nodal or junctional rhythm.

Sinus and junctional rhythms are regular cardiac rhythms. Premature beats alternating with sinus beats constitute a bigeminal rhythm which is a regularly irregular rhythm. Atrial fibrillation is the prototype of an irregularly irregular rhythm.

The P wave is normally associated with the QRS complex that follows it, by a fixed interval. In complete AV block, the P waves and QRS complexes are unrelated to each other and constitute what is referred to as AV dissociation.

The P wave is tall, peaked in right atrial enlargement, broad, notched in left atrial enlargement and absent in atrial flutter and fibrillation. Inverted P waves are observed in junctional rhythm. The P wave is variable in morphology is case of multifocal atrial tachycardia.

The PR interval is prolonged in case of first degree AV block due to rheumatic fever or drugs that block the AV node. The PR interval is shortened in case of a junctional rhythm or in the presence of a preexcitation syndrome.

Potential abnormalities of the QRS complex are variation in height, width, shape and the axis. Tall complexes are seen in ventricular hypertrophy while low-voltage complexes are observed in pericardial effusion. Wide QRS complexes occur in bundle branch block, conduction defect and the WPW syndrome. Alteration in the shape of the QRS complex is in the form of deep S waves or prominent Q waves. There may be rightward or leftward deviation of the QRS axis.

Depression of the ST segment lacks specificity and can occur due to myocardial ischemia, drug effect or an electrolyte abnormality. Elevation of the ST segment is often due to acute myocardial infarction and sometimes due to acute pericarditis or early repolarization.

The QT interval can be prolonged due to a variety of congenital and acquired causes. Similarly, shortening of the QT interval may occur due to a drug effect or an electrolyte imbalance.

Inversion of the T wave, like depression of the ST segment, can occur due to a variety of myocardial and metabolic causes. Tall and peaked T waves are observed during the hyperacute phase of myocardial infarction and in hyperkalemia.

Finally, the U wave may be either prominent or inverted. Prominent U waves are seen in hypokalemia and in patients on digitalis therapy. Inverted U waves are a feature of ischemic heart disease as well as left ventricular diastolic overload.

ECG REPORT

NAME............AGE............SEX............ID.........DATE............

Rate: 72 beats per minute
Rhythm: Sinus arrhythmia
P wave: P. pulmonale
PR interval: 0.18 seconds
QRS complex:

Width   0.10 seconds
Height   Deep Q waves in leads L_1 & V_6
Axis   –30° ; left axis deviation
ST segment: 2 mm depression leads V_4, V_5, V_6
T wave: Low to inverted in leads V_5, V_6
U wave: Prominent in anterior leads

CONCLUSIONS :
1. ECG is within normal limits
   Or
2. ECG is consistent with lateral wall infarction
   Or
3. Abnormal ECG suggestive of lateral infarction

REMARKS :
1. Suggested serial recordings
2. Suggested exercise stress test
3. Suggested repeat in deep inspiration.

ABSENCE OF HEART DISEASE

Normal Subjects
- Sinus arrhythmia
- Incomplete RBBB
- Minor axis deviation
- Upsloping ST depression
- T wave inversion in aVR and V_1
- Supraventricular extrasystole

Athletic built
- Sinus bradycardia
- Sinus arrhythmia
- Junctional rhythm
- First degree AV block
- Wandering pacemaker
- Tall R waves, deep Q waves
- Upsloping ST segment elevation
- Tall and symmetrical T waves.

CONGENITAL HEART DISEASE

Atrial septal defect
- Incomplete RBBB
- Right atrial hypertrophy

Ventricular septal defect
- Biventricular hypertrophy

Right ventricular hypertrophy
- Fallot's tetralogy
- Pulmonary stenosis
- Eisenmenger's syndrome

Left ventricular hypertrophy
- Aortic stenosis
- Coarctation of aorta
- Patent ductus arteriosus
- Hypertrophic cardiomyopathy.

VALVULAR HEART DISEASE

Mitral stenosis
- Atrial fibrillation
- P. mitrale in sinus rhythm
- Right ventricular hypertrophy

Mitral regurgitation
- Atrial fibrillation
- P. mitrale in sinus rhythm
- Left ventricular diastolic overload

Mitral valve prolapse
- Sinus tachycardia
- Premature beats
- T wave inversion in inferior leads
- ST depression in precordial leads

Aortic stenosis
- Left bundle branch block
- Left ventricular hypertrophy
- Left ventricular strain pattern

Aortic regurgitation
- Left anterior hemiblock
- Left ventricular diastolic overload

CORONARY ARTERY DISEASE

Myocardial ischemia
- T wave inversion
- ST segment depression
- Prolonged QT interval

Myocardial infarction
- Sinus tachycardia
- Deep Q waves
- Low R wave height
- T wave inversion
- ST segment elevation
- Ventricular premature beats.

MYOCARDIAL DISEASE

Acute myocarditis
- Sinus tachycardia
- Wide QRS complexes
- QRS electrical alternans
- Prolonged QT interval
- Ventricular arrhythmias

Acute rheumatic fever
- Sinus tachycardia
- First degree AV block
- T wave flattening/inversion
- ST segment depression/elevation

Dilated cardiomyopathy
- Sinus tachycardia
- Bundle branch block
- Left anterior hemiblock
- Reduced QRS complexes
- Ventricular tachyarrhythmias

Hypertrophic cardiomyopathy
- Left anterior hemiblock
- Left ventricular hypertrophy

- Deep T wave inversion
- Prolonged QT interval.

PERICARDIAL DISEASE

Acute pericarditis
- Sinus tachycardia
- Upright T waves
- Concave ST elevation
- PR segment depression

Pericardial effusion
- Sinus tachycardia
- Low QRS voltage
- Electrical alternans
- Nonspecific T inversion.

PULMONARY DISEASE

Pulmonary embolism
- Sinus tachycardia
- Atrial fibrillation
- P. pulmonale
- $S_1Q_{III}T_{III}$ pattern
- Right axis deviation
- Clockwise rotation
- Right bundle branch block
- Right ventricular hypertrophy

Chronic pulmonary disease
- Sinus tachycardia
- Atrial fibrillation
- P. pulmonale
- Right axis deviation
- Right bundle branch block
- Right ventricular hypertrophy
- Nonprogression of the R wave.

INDEX

Page numbers followed by *f* refer to figure and *t* refer to table